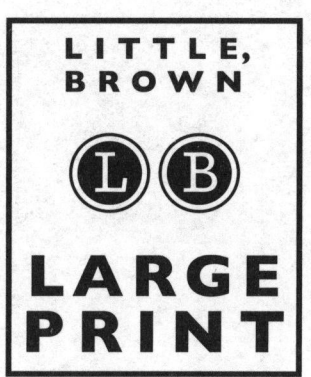

YOU WITH THE SAD EYES

A Memoir

CHRISTINA APPLEGATE

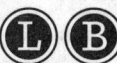

LITTLE, BROWN AND COMPANY

LARGE PRINT EDITION

Author's Note: This is true to what I believe happened. I have changed some names and descriptions. And I have reconstructed dialogue to the best of my recollection and reordered or combined the sequence of some events. Others who were present might recall things differently. But this is my story.

Copyright © 2026 by Christina Applegate

Hachette Book Group supports the right to free expression and the value of copyright. The purpose of copyright is to encourage writers and artists to produce the creative works that enrich our culture.

The scanning, uploading, and distribution of this book without permission is a theft of the author's intellectual property. If you would like permission to use material from the book (other than for review purposes), please contact permissions@hbgusa.com. Thank you for your support of the author's rights.

Little, Brown and Company
Hachette Book Group
1290 Avenue of the Americas, New York, NY 10104
littlebrown.com

First Edition: March 2026

Little, Brown and Company is a division of Hachette Book Group, Inc. The Little, Brown name and logo are trademarks of Hachette Book Group, Inc.

The publisher is not responsible for websites (or their content) that are not owned by the publisher.

The Hachette Speakers Bureau provides a wide range of authors for speaking events. To find out more, go to hachettespeakersbureau.com or email hachettespeakers@hbgusa.com.

Little, Brown and Company books may be purchased in bulk for business, educational, or promotional use. For information, please contact your local bookseller or the Hachette Book Group Special Markets Department at special.markets@hbgusa.com.

Photo insert credits: page 7 courtesy of Sam Sarkar; page 14 (top) courtesy of Adir Abergel; page 15 (both) courtesy of Adir Abergel. All other photographs courtesy of the author.

Reproduction of Andrew Wyeth's CHRISTINA'S WORLD © 2025 Wyeth Foundation for American Art / Artists Rights Society (ARS), New York. Digital Image © The Museum of Modern Art/Licensed by SCALA / Art Resource, NY.

ISBN 9780316594929 (hardcover) / 9780316601665 (large print) / 9780316604000 (signed edition) / 9780316604673 (B&N signed edition)
Library of Congress Control Number: 2025950661

Printing 1, 2025

LSC-C

Printed in the United States of America

This is for Sadie. Everything I do is for Sadie. Writing this book is for Sadie. These next words are for Sadie:

My darling child, you are my reason, my season, and my lifetime.

CONTENTS

Prologue 5

ONE: Star, Fucker! 19
TWO: LaLa Land 40
THREE: The Bathroom Floor 60
FOUR: Quit 87
FIVE: *Married...with Children* 113
SIX: Nostradamus 145
SEVEN: The Orange Curtains 178
EIGHT: Hawaii 207
NINE: Filthy McNasty 218
TEN: Red Wedding 231
ELEVEN: Bing Bang Boom 243
TWELVE: Metatarsal #5 252

Contents

THIRTEEN: Kibitz Kismet 271

FOURTEEN: Right Action for Women 285

FIFTEEN: Pinch 302

SIXTEEN: Who Do I Think I Am? 311

SEVENTEEN: *Dead To Me* 326

EIGHTEEN: The Lady in the Bathtub from *The Shining* 348

Acknowledgments 369

YOU WITH THE SAD EYES

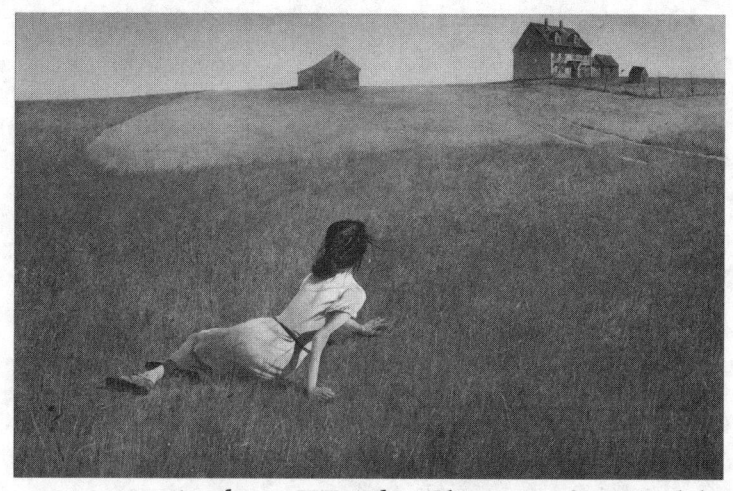
Andrew Wyeth, Christina's World, *1948*

Christina has a bonny face
Nobody knows the secret place
    Nancy Priddy, "Christina's World," 1968

"What we all want is someone who will accept us for what we are and what we have become."
    From my diary, Wednesday, August 6, 2008

PROLOGUE

My mom always told me that I was a sad little girl.

"You were just born that way," she'd say.

But I actually don't believe that's true. I was introduced to the weight of the world much too early on in life. I think being left by my father and growing up in a household that was abusive and scary and awful may have loaned me those sad eyes. Even if I hadn't admitted it to myself, my sad eyes had been revealing the true me all along.

Looking back, I guess I've faked it until I made it my whole life. When you've been through the kinds of things I've been through, you have to get good at hiding behind a persona, and my Christina Applegate persona was successful, especially in shielding me from having to face the past.

That was then. But now? I embrace my sad eyes—I've earned them.

In my public life, I've played the character "Christina Applegate" for so long, since I was a very young child. The comic actor, the serious actor, the all-singing, all-dancing, ultimate performer, the good talk show interview—I was all those things. I even wrote a paper in school professing myself a "triple threat" and saying I wanted to be Meryl Streep.

That person is unrecognizable to me now.

I am not Christina Applegate.

Recently, I noticed that a dear friend of mine had me listed as "Christina Applegate" in her phone.

"Take that out," I said. "And don't you ever call me by those two names together." It took her a moment, but she understood.

Anyone who truly knows me knows I am not Christina Applegate.

I was never, ever that person. Whenever I hear "Christina Applegate" I get spine tingles, and not in a good way. Those two words together do not denote the secret place, the center of my soul, the real me.

Instead, there's one nickname I save for my true essence. Usually, I don't want the world to see who I really am, so I have kept it secret. But when those closest to me use my nickname, just two short syllables, I feel they know me in the deepest and most beautiful way.

I promise by the end of this book you'll know those two syllables, too, and not just in name. I'll finally reveal every reason for those sad eyes, will describe the full spectrum of a life seen through them — the good, the bad, the ups, the downs, the everything.

It's not a process I'm looking forward to, being that vulnerable. But I want to reveal who I am, fully, for the first time. Maybe I don't even know who that is, but hey, I have nothing left to lose.

In 2021, I was diagnosed with multiple sclerosis. MS attacks your nervous system and slows down your functions — your respiratory system, your organs, everything. The disease eats away at all the things we take for granted. Some of us with MS have a raft of pain; some don't. I have a lot of it. When I wake up, I often can't get my arm to move far enough to grab the cup of water by my bed or my phone from its charger. I have infusions every six months to slow the disease's progress, but those infusions kill all the B cells in my body, making me prone to infection. My stomach frequently slows to a halt, leaving me to regularly rush to the emergency room in agony. Most days, simply walking across the room feels like scaling a mountain.

One of the worst side effects of the illness is the exhaustion. It feels as though I've been on a three-day-long sleepless bender, but no bender for me — that's how I feel after a *good* night's sleep. Hence all the time

I spend on and in bed, snuggled up against Jake Ryan, which is what I call my heating pad. A sidenote that if you were born in the seventies, as I was, *Sixteen Candles* was the shit. In the last moment of the movie, Jake Ryan, wearing bad jeans in front of a red Porsche, looks at Sam Baker (played by Molly Ringwald) and says, "Yeah, you." If you don't know what that means, put this book down right now and go watch the movie. It's much more uplifting.

As you may be catching on, on the back of that diagnosis and the symptoms I face, I no longer care what I say or how I come across or how it makes anyone feel. I don't have patience for bullshit anymore, no patience for things that are meaningless or merely "extra." Add to that, I don't have room for inauthenticity or hidden meanings. There's no longer subtext when I speak. Everything I say is true, and unadorned, and real.

This is new for me, as I've always been a private person. When I was growing up, we didn't have trolls, cellphones, social media. Instead, we just had the Z Channel, which was famous for airing the seminal music video, "Brass in Pocket" by the Pretenders. There was no MTV, no Bravo, no *Real Housewives*—just that video airing once in a while in between televised movies. I didn't live a public life the way celebrities have to now. At the time, everything was more private.

In many ways, I know I seem to have lived a perfect

life, and I've been told that this has inspired some people to look up to me. The truth is, I never felt seen. Just as I know that so many people who have suffered in different ways haven't felt seen either. I succeeded in life despite what I went through, but it's time to tell the truth, even if while writing this I feel like I'm giving a TED talk. I promise, I'm not!

And it's not just because I'm no longer working. Sure, there's no one breathing down my neck to represent their business or their movie or their TV show, things I've had to represent, usually willingly and passionately, for almost fifty years. It goes deeper. I've become an honesty missile. When your physical situation deteriorates, and your life shrinks to the size of a California king, suddenly all the things you thought were important shift, too. The truth clarifies, like a camera lens slowly focusing.

I know it's a cliché that clowns are sad, but my outward success and humor masked a tough life, and an abiding sense that I wasn't good enough. I hid all that for the good of whatever movie or TV show or play I was representing. Now, those days are gone. I have one friend who insists I'll work again, but he doesn't see the full extent of my pain.

In fact, my body has let me down so much that I've taken to naming the various parts so I can yell at them. My entire body is Sylvia, so if I have weird things going on, my friends will yell, "Stop, Sylvia, stop it!"

Sometimes I get weird shakes in Barbara (my right arm), and once in a while Stanley (left arm) joins in.

My right leg is Meghan Markle.

Don't ask.

My left leg is Tootie, from *The Facts of Life*.

My gallbladder is named Gail, my liver Olivia. My kidneys are Calliope. I haven't named my intestines yet, and I probably should because I'm mad at them all the time.

Stacey's a bitch, but Staceys are always bitches, aren't they? Stacey is my stomach.

When Barbara and Stanley and Meghan and Tootie and Gail and Olivia and Calliope and Stacey are doing weird things, I try to talk to them, and because I have a disease of the nervous system, it's almost like they listen. When I was first diagnosed, Barbara would shake constantly, and one of my friends, Carolyn, would yell, "Barbara! Be quiet!" Sometimes it would help.

My brain has a name, too: Stuart, aka Fucking Asshole.

This disease has robbed me of who I am, has robbed me of my life, of the things I loved. I was invincible. I loved running. I loved Peloton, I played tennis, and I loved—I mean really loved—to dance.

I want to pick up the guitar over there by the wall,

but my hands cramp. I used to love saying to Sadie, my amazing daughter, "Yes, of course I'll take you wherever you want to go in the car." Now, I often can't drive her anywhere.

But I like to watch TV—the worse the better, usually reality shows like *Real Housewives*—because with TV I get to escape. I don't have to think. I don't want narratives, art, series in which you invest in some antihero across seven brilliant seasons. I want rich women screaming at each other.

I keep the TV on twenty-four hours a day because without it the quiet is so loud in my head I can't bear it.

Would I have wanted it this way, to have everything stripped away? Did I envision finally arriving at a place of raw honesty about my life, and that would be a *good* thing? Fuck no. I want to work and dance and take Sadie everywhere, but being forced into this home-based life has stripped away my last vestiges of reserve. It has afforded me time and space to look back on my life and take stock of it for the first time. Alongside the need to confront the truth and enormity of all that I have lived through, a beautiful thing emerged: I have started to make a little sense of it, to understand what happened, see patterns, discover meaning, find the love and acceptance and healing in it, and start to forgive myself, to give my young self, especially, some slack for all the bad decisions and self-destructive behaviors.

* * *

In my closet there is a locked box of all my journals from the age of thirteen to the time I stopped wanting to write. I had told my best friend and godmother of my child, Rachel, that when I die, she may open the box. I never thought it would be opened before I was gone.

Lucky you—the box is open. I'm going to extensively quote from those journals. I've kept meticulous records, all too aware that those pages were the only place I could share the unfiltered truth.

I recently showed my daughter the diary I wrote when I was thirteen, and she said, "You were *fucked up*." I mean, my mom was in an abusive relationship when I was little. I gave my first blow job at thirteen. I was madly in love with Johnny Depp at fifteen. I was plagued by disordered eating and self-loathing from my teens on. It's all in there. All the way up to me having cancer.

I'm finally free to reveal the true me, and in doing so, I hope in some small way you might be able to come to terms with some of your past, too. Just because life has sometimes been tough—and maybe at certain points it even felt impossible—that doesn't mean we have to wallow in the darkness or be stymied by our histories. I'm here to tell you that despite how dark it gets, there's a lot to gain from mining one's past for meaning.

One of the things I've begun to see more clearly through my newfound freedom is that I'm a survivor. Given everything, I really shouldn't still be here. But underneath all that Susan Applebee (what a woman in Santa Monica once insisted my name was) BS was a radically honest, genuine person who formed real connections, lifelong connections. I'm a good fucking friend, and this world needs more good friends. I survived it all thanks to an abiding passion to overcome, and an unwavering belief in myself, a belief that whatever the world threw at me — and man, it threw a lot, and it's still throwing — I had to get to the other side of something. I want you to know that the other side is worth the fight. That you are always worth fighting for, and that you are never alone in your fight.

This book is a witness to that survival, and all the things I endured that I never told anyone because it was all too heartbreaking: the good stuff, the terrible stuff, the hilarious stuff, the shitty sad stuff. I have a degenerative disease that has probably ended my performing career, and without that, what is there to hide? And I truly believe that living in truth will liberate all of us: you, me, everyone.

I've packed a lot into these fifty-something years. For a long time, it felt impossible to find the meaning in everything I've been through, but I have come to understand that we ultimately get to choose what defines us—and the working through of that will be what drives the narrative of this book. I will detail what that pain has taught me, and in turn, what it has allowed me to release. I want readers to understand what each of us facing our pain can learn from getting on and getting through.

Many of the revelations about my childhood and much of my life will shock a lot of people. It's scary—not going to lie—to finally decide to tell it all. Some days, when I open up the box in my closet and turn the pages of the many diaries I keep locked in there, I want to shut it all away as quickly as I opened it. My journals are a contemporary record of a girl becoming a woman and having to fight for every scrap of love she received, and sometimes it's just too much to read back across those years. I want to save the six-year-old me, the eleven-year-old, the nineteen-year-old, the thirty-two-year-old... But I guess I already saved her, a little bit, at least, because here she is, sharing her most intimate moments from forty years of journaling, all in the hope of showing you that you don't have to feel alone—you too can find your way, you too can survive. Hell, you too can flourish as I once did, before MS forced me into this prison of a bed.

In my ongoing effort to survive, it's imperative for me to share my life with you. I hope in doing so that you can know you're not alone, that someone else has had to survive, and has done so while making people laugh.

There is always light, always, and the deeper I dig into my past, the more good I'm unearthing, the more positives I have uncovered, things I can hold on to on the hardest days. I'll tell a ton of stories about *Married...with Children,* about *Anchorman,* about *Sweet Charity,* about *Dead to Me,* and about the incredible people who've been in my life, from my mother to my daughter and so many in between.

There will be happy chapters about my wonderful friends and life, about my daughter's amazing father and my husband (our love story spans a couple of lifetimes). Sadie, my brilliant daughter, will be a constant character, too, wandering in and out of the book. There will even be an account of my trawlerman boyfriend who is long gone but who now literally haunts my house, and there will be writing about my illnesses: my breast cancer and my MS. I'll show how my mother got past her addictions. I'll talk about my faith, and I'll talk about (and probably *to*) God, and about karma, and all the things in between, all the things that I've learned that have made me a survivor, things I want to share with readers to perhaps help them survive, too. Because everybody has something, and everyone needs to be seen, this book is my way of seeing, of sharing the details of my life so that others can move forward in theirs.

I've called it survival, but it's really more like *freedom*. By working through it all on the page, I intend to release myself fully into a life of acceptance, hope, and joy.

Of course, none of us turn out perfect. We're always evolving, we're always changing. I will work through much of my life in this book, but the true beauty of it is that I'm in my fifties and I still don't know what the hell is happening. What you're about to read is an account of something that I've only recently started to come to terms with. I may never fully do so. I can't reshape this life into some perfect story with a cherry on top. It was not a perfect life — far from it.

None of our stories are perfect. Every person has a level of sadness. This is just an account of mine.

I don't have the answers, but I do have a story.

I'll still be pissed off, of course, but there's a river of love that runs through this house these days. People come by, sit on the end of the bed, and we connect and reminisce and most of all we share love and hope. This book aims to capture all that.

In every instance the pain will be matched by the joy, the losses mitigated by the extraordinary life I've been so lucky to lead. Not even my best friends who sit by my bedside know the full details; sure, they know some of it, but even then, they often think I'm making it up because it is all so unbelievable.

We find the joy where we can. For me, most often

it's in the form of a teenage daughter who makes everything better.

So no, this book won't be like some big violin scratching for my life. I'm still pretty funny. But it will be real.

So here I am.

Real me.

Lots to say.

ONE

STAR, FUCKER!

The line from Grauman's Chinese Theatre went all the way around the block. This is Los Angeles, California, 1977. Teens, preteens, parents, nerds, punks, space cadets, hippies, peaceniks—it seemed like the whole, spaced-out, Jimmy Carter, tube-socked world was here, May 25, the opening day of a movie called *Star Wars*.

Already, even before the first notes of John Williams's legendary score, the world had lost its mind to Princess Leia and Luke and R2-D2 and Darth Vader. Even though I wouldn't be six years old until the end of the year, there I was, just as nuts as everyone else— I couldn't *wait* to see it. The May warmth bounced off Hollywood Boulevard; intermittent shade beckoned us, and we huddled in it whenever we could as the line inched forward. We drudged forward patiently, but we jiggled about in excitement, too, praying we'd make it to the box office before the whole thing sold out.

I wasn't alone. Occasionally I'd look up at my mom and smile at her. She'd smile back (her blissful grin was then brought to you by Valium). My mother was, and is, a beautiful woman. She always smelled of rose perfume, and in the evenings, I loved lying in her lap, safe in the scent of her, listening to the house finches and mockingbirds and a distant great horned owl hooting out there in the dark of Laurel Canyon, where we lived.

I always felt safe with my mom. She was my entire world. We were alone together. This was not what she'd envisioned for her life, a single mother with a five-year-old kid, short on cash, her musical career stalled. But here she was, and here I was, and there, soon, would be Luke and Leia and Chewbacca and R2-D2 and a distant, heavy-voiced man who would turn out to be an absentee father...

We didn't come down to the bustle of Hollywood all that often. We lived in Laurel Canyon on Lookout Mountain (which felt many more than the two miles from Hollywood it was), in a 750-square-foot row house.

That day in 1977, Mom and I had driven down the

winding mountain and made a sharp left into Hollywood in our beaten-down Chevy Nova, eager to be transported into outer space. But before I could be dispatched into a galaxy far, far away, something else, something even more magical, attracted my attention: everywhere I looked on that burning sidewalk there were *stars* built into the concrete.

"Mama, what are all those stars for?" I asked.

"They're for famous performers," my mom, herself a singer, said.

"What did they do? Was it good or was it bad? Who are these people, Mama?"

As my mother tried to explain, I could feel something sparking in me, indistinctly at first, and then, catching hold, like a wildfire. My mom and I had slowly inched to the front of Grauman's, to the spot where you can reach down and put your hands in handprints and your feet in footprints of famous performers, and I reached down to put my little five-and-a-half-year-old hands into Jack Nicholson's imprint, which he'd made in June 1974. (I had no idea that one day I'd be ineffectually flirting with him in an audition for a movie role.)

I distinctly remember thinking, even at five years old, *This is* magic! *These people will be here* forever.

A child's mind can conceive of the beauty of forever. Especially when the present presses hard, like a burden.

* * *

That child's mind had already had to come to terms with too many burdens.

I was raised in Laurel Canyon, which, though once the epicenter of a legendary arts scene, had become, by the time I showed up, at least, a different kind of place.

The original Laurel Canyon scene had developed in the mid- to late sixties—back then, houses in the Canyon had been both affordable and gratifyingly hidden away above the thrum of Sunset Boulevard and Hollywood, and a host of musicians and artists and actors had made the place their creative home. Even today when you turn off Sunset or Hollywood Boulevard and head north into Laurel Canyon, whispers of something ethereal and magical and inspiring seem to drift from the laurels and the eucalyptus.

The streets are narrow and winding, perched on the side of steep hills, which are themselves discreet, peaceful, cool, and shaded. Back in the late sixties, this was the land of Joni Mitchell's Trina and her wampum beads, where music poured down the Canyon, "cats and babies" all around the women's feet, characters wrapped "in songs and gypsy shawls." Mitchell lived here for a while, as did Neil Young, Carole King, Jackson Browne, David Crosby, Stephen

Stills, Graham Nash, Mama Cass, and James Taylor, and so did Frank Zappa and his Girls Together Outrageously (GTOs) cohort, who all lived together for a time at 2401 Laurel Canyon Boulevard, opposite Houdini's house. Mitchell and Nash, the ultimate Canyon couple, famously bought a vase on Ventura Boulevard in the Valley one morning and by the afternoon Nash had written "Our House" about the vase and the house the two artists shared on Lookout Mountain, half a mile from where I would grow up. The power of the Canyon's creative inspiration could foster a classic song and some attendant wild behavior, but it could also cause these artists to lose their minds — Jackson Browne is on the record as saying, "What was happening in Laurel Canyon was the universe cracking open and revealing its secrets."

But by the late sixties something else was cracking open — a darker edge to the Canyon was appearing. The Manson murders had taken place in August 1969 a couple of canyons over, at 10050 Cielo Drive in Benedict Canyon, about three miles as the raven flies from Laurel. After that, Michelle Phillips of the Mamas and the Papas said she started carrying a gun in her purse when she walked the winding Laurel Canyon streets. Joni Mitchell and Graham Nash broke up. Folk music stalwarts became mega pop superstars and moved away to places with gates and security. The drugs were maturing from weed to cocaine and heroin. Murders would come to our part of Laurel Canyon, too.

And into this dying scene moved Nancy Priddy and Bob Applegate.

Nancy Priddy was born in South Bend, Indiana, on January 22, 1941, the very day the Andrews Sisters recorded "Boogie Woogie Bugle Boy" and the Americans captured the Libyan stronghold of Tobruk. Later, when the war was over, and when my mother had graduated (from Northwestern with a degree in English), she moved on her own — like so many hippie-folkies — to New York City's version of Laurel Canyon, Greenwich Village, where, *un*like many of the other transplants who barely bathed, she turned into a stunning hippie sexpot. She sang with the house band at the historic Greenwich Village folk club the Bitter End (there she is, her hair dyed black and in a chic bob, bottom right, on the cover of a Bitter End Singers' album from 1964) and with Leonard Cohen (you can hear her backing vocals on classics like "Suzanne" and "So Long, Marianne"), among others.

In 1968, my mother released a beautiful album of her own called *You've Come This Way Before,* produced by the legendary Phil Ramone. On that record's cover she's sitting on cobblestones and looking wistfully over her right shoulder, her long ginger hair cascading just so. She might well be thinking about Stephen Stills in that photo—the title song is about him. In the late sixties he and my mom had fallen into a passionate relationship. They lived together for a while in New York at around the time one of Stephen's bands, Buffalo Springfield, was recording his seminal song "For What It's Worth (Stop, Hey What's That Sound)," which he wrote about the L.A. Sunset Strip curfew riots of late 1966. Stephen would come back to the house he shared with my mother and complain that he was singing flat, or say ridiculous things like "This song's *horrible*," even though it would become one of the greatest songs of the 1960s counterculture scene. Stephen would later become my godfather. I call him Uncle Dadu (Uncle Daddy), but that comes later.

At about the same time, there was a guy named Bob Applegate hanging around, a music promoter who would eventually become a producer at Casablanca Records. In the pictures of him from back then, a wide, smiling, warm face peers out, usually above a wide-lapelled, open-necked shirt, gaudy chain, and three-piece suit, as he hobnobs with music industry people or leans over a mixing board in a studio. This obviously charming man desperately wanted to date the enchanting Nancy Priddy.

One weekend, Stephen Stills was supposed to call my mom and didn't. Nancy Priddy was so pissed off that she went on a revenge date with Bob Applegate. As the story goes, Stephen hadn't called my mother because he was deep in a secret affair with Judy Collins, a relationship that birthed yet another classic track, "Suite: Judy Blue Eyes," one of the best songs that was ever recorded. So it all worked out right in the end, I guess: the world got "Judy Blue Eyes," and my dad got my mom, and thereafter, *moi*.

After that date my mom and dad fell super crazy in love, moved west, and lived together in Laurel Canyon on Lookout Mountain, where all the doors were still open, where musicians wandered up and down the streets in their bathrobes, went in and out of each other's homes to play music, write classic songs, smoke pot, all in that free-love, happy-happy, goody-goody kind of way—a place where everybody had their legs spread, including the men. The 1960s gave way to the 1970s, and it seemed like everybody was still doing everybody.

And then sometime early in 1971, Nancy Priddy fell pregnant. With the jasmine night-blooming across the Canyon, my mother bloomed, too, until spring became summer became fall, and it was Thursday, November 25—actual swear-to-God Thanksgiving Day—and instead of gobbling down turkey and gravy, my parents were rushing to a hospital in the Little Armenia section of Los Angeles. I was born at 5:45 p.m., in what is now a huge Scientology building (its address is 1403 North L. Ron Hubbard Way), but which at the time was the Cedars of Lebanon medical building. As an aside, my dear friend was born the day before Thanksgiving, and her parents gave her the middle name Cranberry. I guess I dodged a bullet with Christina—lord knows I could have been Turkey Gravy Applegate, or worse, Stuffing Applegate.

My mother was thirty years old when I showed up. Thanksgiving Day had delivered her a child, a girl she did indeed name Christina, after her favorite painting, Andrew Wyeth's 1948 masterpiece, *Christina's World*.

It's almost too strange a coincidence, given everything that's happened to me in the past few years, that *Christina's World* depicts a neighbor of Wyeth, one Anna Christina Olson, who suffered from some kind of degenerative muscle condition. Ms. Olson always refused a wheelchair, choosing instead to crawl. Wyeth once said of the painting, "The challenge to me was to do justice to her extraordinary conquest of a life which most people would consider hopeless."

And here I am, with MS, some days feeling hopeless, but still crawling my way forward, still in my own extraordinary conquest of a life. My mother called me Christina—nothing is an accident—after a girl who couldn't walk.

Now, five decades later, some days I can't walk either. But no wheelchair for me. Instead, here I am, crawling around through my weeds. Back then, too, my mother was about to fall into deep weeds, weeds it would take her decades to crawl through until she made her own kind of escape.

By my bedside I keep a large, battered, brown leather photo album that my father created back in 1972. At the start of the album, he has written his daughter a letter.

Christina,

Today, May 26th, year 1972, you & I took our first walk together. You had been in New York & New Jersey for the past two months. You were placed in my backpack & off we went.
Now at the beginning of our walk you weren't too happy and had been suffering with your first teeth. As we walked along, I placed my finger in your mouth. That seemed to do the trick, and you were suddenly fast asleep. We walked up around the back roads of our home, to the top of a big hill. There we sat for a while, looking out over the countryside. You were still asleep, but I knew you were content with the situation. We started back down the hill only to be stopped by a beautiful

brown and white bird who so proudly sang for us. As we walked a BIG German shepherd said, "Hello," and guess what? That's right, you opened your big blue eyes, but only for a moment, then back to sleep. When we arrived by home, you were, shall we say, sort of awake, sort of asleep. And that was our first walk together. It was a happy moment.

> *Daddy*
> *PS. Six months old... wow.*

My father has filled the subsequent pages with pictures of me, of him, of me and him, and of me and my mother. He has decorated the pages with pressed flowers, and with pictures of flowers and children. As I turn the pages, I see my father on a snowy mountainside; there he is again, smoking a joint (he's written "Peace!" on that photo—of course he has). There I am in a red outfit and white Mary Janes; sitting on his lap on a carousel horse; again on his lap as he plays a piano, no shirt (him, not me). There I am in my mother's arms, and at a birthday party; in a stroller, or peering in surprise at the flash from a photo booth, my father's huge beard scratching my baby face.

But there are no pictures of me and my parents together. Instead, there are pictures of my father with a different partner, a different family.

* * *

In his note, my father references a trip east to New York and New Jersey. Right after I showed up that Thanksgiving in 1971, my paternal grandparents asked to see me—they lived in Lawrenceville, New Jersey. So when my mom went to New York for work, I went to see my grandparents.

In New York, my mom was to tape an episode of *Days of Our Lives,* and I was in the episode, too. I was three months old. The episode, number 1,597, aired on March 7, 1972. In it, I play baby Burt Grizzell, "son" of Mrs. Grizzell, played by my mother. (I would be invited back for a subsequent episode, though without my mother this time, and still a boy.) Mom and I also did a Playtex Nurser commercial together, in which my mother is bottle-feeding me with a Playtex collapsible bottle while saying, "What a difference! Now she has less gas . . . because natural nipples mean less air in her tummy!"

(Three and a half decades later I would write in my diary, "Sat up again. Sponge bath humiliation. So gassy. That was funny. Walked to the window." This was four days after the double mastectomy that saved my life.)

Two months later, my father wrote another letter to me in that album.

> *Oh my child we are together again, only to find that we shall be together always. We are in Big Sur now, and you are 8 months old—wow! Can you believe it? What is Big Sur, you asked—well, it's a paradise for those who understand, those who wish to get back to the basics, but wish to grow...*

That reference to Big Sur hangs heavy. When my mother called my father to say she was heading home from that first trip to the East Coast, his two-word reply devastated her and set in motion a chain of terrible events for me and my mom, events whose ripples still move through both of our lives.

"We're on our way home," my mom said.

"So *soon*?" my dad said.

He really didn't need to say anything else.

There is a photo from that time that haunts me now because it presages so much of what was to come. In it, my heavily bearded father is sitting cross-legged in a white sleeveless tee, head shaved, at the foot of what looks like two redwoods. This is him at Big Sur—it appears he's communing with something, almost Buddha-like, the once-slick music executive in a suit now replaced by this uncompromising figure in combat boots. He looks more like he's spent time in San Quentin than Monterey County.

With those two words—"So *soon*?"—Dad headed

away from Nancy Priddy, away from his newborn, to make a new life in Big Sur on the Pacific Coast, six hours north of Laurel Canyon. When we arrived home, he was gone.

My father never came back.

For us, it was a disaster; for him, it would prove to be a kismet move. On the first day he got to Big Sur, a woman staying at the same rooming house told him that she could feel his presence in the building. Family lore goes that she wandered downstairs and said to Bob Applegate, "Are you a Scorpio?"

"Yes, I am," he said, and that was about all it took — something ignited, and they were together from that moment on, early in 1972, right up until Tuesday, March 18, 2025, at 4:59 a.m., when my father died.

What to make of my father's abandonment of me and my mother? He always claimed that he was convinced that my mom was continuing to have an affair with Stephen Stills while she was pregnant with me, but anyone who's ever been pregnant knows that the last thing you want to do is have sex with someone who's *not* the father — if you want to have sex at all. I think it was simply my dad's way of justifying leaving us.

There is a third letter to me in that photo album.

You with the Sad Eyes

Christina's World by Daddy

> *We've been here now for 2 days. You, my darling, have caused quite a rush, not only for me but for everyone who touches you. These two days, as the few times we have spent together before, have been the highest, and most peaceful and fulfilling days of life.*
>
> *Later tonight if it's okay with you, we shall sit by the fire and together become one. So high — you make me so high!*

I don't think I was the only thing making my father high back then. My father was doing a lot of acid in the early 1970s, and his brain seemed in chaos. Acid will force a mind into telling lies to itself, lies like the one about my mother continuing to have a relationship with Stephen Stills. They were lies my father believed, and lies that crushed my mother and would eventually confuse and hurt his new daughter, when she became old enough to know that her father was gone.

But there was so much more to my father's life than LSD-generated stories. And it all began long before I showed up. When I uncovered the real story, everything changed, but that would take me another thirty years.

* * *

Bob was gone, into a new relationship, a new orbit, so high, so high, and my mother and I were left entirely alone. I went to Big Sur as a little baby a few times, until my father and his new wife moved first to Burbank, in the Valley, and then to Woodland Hills, out on the 101 near Calabasas. I was court-ordered to go to his new house, which had a pool, at least, every other weekend for years — I hated it, but I'll admit I loved the pool and idyllic setting. My father was by now back in the music business full-time, and things had gone well enough that he drove a Mercedes.

Mom and I had our beaten-down Nova and lived in a little row house.

It wasn't entirely my dad's fault that I didn't like visiting. I just wanted to be home with my mom. I vividly remember each time we'd head back on the 101. The second I would see the communications tower above the Mulholland Tennis Club, which signals the high point of Laurel Canyon, I'd get giddy — great fluttering butterflies in my stomach — because I knew I was going to see her.

It was just the two of us, Nancy Priddy and her daughter, Christina Applegate, alone together in Laurel Canyon. When I would come home, I'd get the same feeling as when we would go to Magic Mountain — I'd see the waterslide on the hill and know I was close to one of my favorite places in all of Southern California.

My mom was always my Magic Mountain, too.

Back in 1968, in the gatefold of her album, my mother had written a short essay to introduce herself. This is how it begins.

> One day a lyricist and good friend of mine said to me, "Nancy, why do you always write sad lyrics? You seem to see primarily the negative side of things." Taken back a little, I went home and started reading through the reams of backs of envelopes, scraps of crumpled papers, and an occasional poorly typed piece of onion skin that I had accumulated. What a discovery one can make about oneself. It's not unlike a Rorschach test or finding strange patterns in a collection of doodles.
> What I discovered was not necessarily negativism or sadness, but an obvious quality of disappointment throughout the somewhat subconscious ramblings. I am an Aquarian and have been told that I am the true embodiment of Aquarius—for what

it's worth. It's not negativism, but extreme
positivism that is at the basis of what I
write—an incurable idealism that often
gets rained, snowed, sleeted, and hailed
upon by life.

Three years later, her love affair with my father over, the positivism of the move west and the birth of a child had been utterly subsumed by the rain, snow, sleet, and hail of abandonment.

And so was set a pattern that I too would follow my entire life: I share with my mother an idealism, a positivism, that is so often followed by terrible weather. In thinking back across my life, I have realized that when good things happen to me, as many good things have, they are invariably stalked by darkness, dampened by subsequent tragedies and trauma. My mother wrote, *"I went home and started reading through the reams of backs of envelopes, scraps of crumpled papers, and an occasional poorly typed piece of onion skin... What a discovery one can make about oneself. It's not unlike a Rorschach test or finding strange patterns in a collection of doodles. What I discovered was not necessarily negativism or sadness, but an obvious quality of disappointment."* In my mom's words, I see not only her own foreshadowing of the pain Bob Applegate would bring into her life, but my own story, too. Here I am, looking back through the *"scraps of crumpled papers"* that constitute my own diaries, and I find throughout a similar sense of disappointment.

These days, as I sit on my bed in pain from the MS, my acting and dancing careers over, I think about the moments in my life when wonderful things have been followed by the dreadful. I finally made it to Broadway, only to get a terrible injury; I finally got the role of a lifetime in *Dead to Me,* only to find out I had MS halfway through. This pattern is seemingly a genetic gift from my mother, a woman so haunted by her own disappointments that she chose to highlight them in the sleeve notes to her album.

My father had escaped to chase a different consciousness in Big Sur, away, perhaps, from the shadows he saw in my mother's eyes.

She and I, meanwhile, had to pick up the pieces however best we could. She tried her best to make our odd little house a home, but it was hard. Among its many "charms" was one narrow, three-foot-by-two-foot door near the ceiling that you had to walk up tiny stairs to reach and then crouch through to get to my bedroom, which was itself an illegally converted garage. It also housed for free so many fleas that when I wore white socks to school, there would be hundreds of tiny black dots visible on them.

My mom never made us feel like we were poor, though, whatever she was facing on a daily basis. She certainly never *said* we were poor. The only thing she did say regularly was, "Don't spend your money because you might be poor one day." She taught me the value of things, and I still have those values. That's why to this day I mostly wear secondhand clothing, which is often stuff I stole from set. My mom's words — "Be careful" — ring in my ears.

But it wasn't all bad. We could still drive our Nova down the mountain to the movies, just the two of us. We could join the lines on May 25, 1977, to see the magic of *Star Wars* for the first time. And a five-year-old girl could still dream of a future when she too had a star.

It's no exaggeration to say that from that moment in 1977 onward, my whole goal in life was to get a star on that Walk of Fame. Because if that was to happen — if one day a crowd would gather and watch a star with my name on it be revealed from under a banner — then I'd be on this spinning planet forever. And maybe someday some kid would say, "Who's that, Mommy?" And maybe the mommy gets to explain who I was.

An Oscar would be lovely, but you know what? You win the Oscar, give a six-minute speech, and nobody cares two days later, especially if your speech lasts six minutes just like it inevitably does the first time you give one. You put the naked-man statue in your guest bathroom, and it's over. Ask an Oscar recipient where they keep their trinket and they're likely to have to take a moment to remember exactly where it is.

But a star? Encased in concrete? Assuming no earthquake destroys it, the worst you'd have to deal with would be the traipsing feet of millions of tourists. No one ever forgets where their star resides—everyone knows the exact cross street without hesitation.

So a star became my lofty goal. A star would be *my* Oscar.

TWO

LALA LAND

RECENTLY, I FOUND A photograph taken sometime in the mid-1970s. In it, Stephen Stills—Uncle Dadu—is perched on the arm of a couch in a red shirt; behind him stands my father's stepmother, Olive, and next to him sits my grandfather, Paul Applegate. My mother is also sitting on the couch, with me in a baby bikini leaning over her. And behind her, a man in glasses rests his hands on my mother's shoulders, smiling at the camera as though everything is wonderful in this garden-variety family snap.

I was so shocked when I stumbled on the photo I could barely breathe. I couldn't make sense of it; how was that man in glasses in the same room as my grandfather and his wife? Why was Stephen Stills there? Where was the photograph taken? Who took it? And how, given what I know now, were we all smiling so broadly, so innocently, at the unseen photographer?

Seeing the photo sent me spinning back to those days after my father left. Many of the keys to my life are encapsulated in those months and years; they headline the story I'm telling, reverberate still, make a music I wish I had never heard.

I have a lot of time to think now that I'm basically bedbound. But this photograph... I just can't make sense of it. It has given me a sense of earthmoving, an odd feeling of dislocation, as though my memory of those days is flawed. Again, I have to ask myself: how can what I know to be true be so in opposition to the easy smiles of this family pic? These six people in this picture look like the epitome of a happy family, broad smiles on happy faces, not a care in the world.

A happy family...?

Well, no, I was not raised in a happy family, in a happy place. Generational trauma is a real thing; I am living proof of it. This photograph sits beside my bed, and when I pick it up, beneath it I find a stain on my nightstand as though something altogether too hot has rested there too long.

I found out recently that the photograph was taken in Florida, probably in 1974, when Stephen was making his solo record *Stills,* which the man in glasses, a percussionist, played on, and which was partially recorded at the legendary Criteria Studios in North Miami. My grandparents were there because it was easier for them to visit Florida from New Jersey than to schlep all the way to California.

I stare at the man behind my mother. He's wearing a T-shirt that reads ITALIAN above a fist of power. Behind his head the flash of the camera obscures the photographer. But that flash obscures everything else, too.

At least until now.

The fleas weren't the only vermin in our house on Lookout Mountain. After a couple of years of being alone, my mother invited into our lives a new man, a man who would unironically wear an Italian-power T-shirt and smile for the camera. He was the worst man imaginable.

With my father literally and figuratively out of the picture, my mother—shocked, hurt, lonely, scared, poor, devastated—got incredibly skinny and sick. At around that time, she was introduced to a musician, someone who played percussion for CSNY, the Eagles, the Bee Gees, Jackson Browne, Jimi Hendrix, Janis Joplin, John Lennon, Barbra Streisand, Eric Clapton, Whitney Houston, Herbie Hancock—the list goes on and on.

This was the man in the photograph.

Sometimes in books people fudge the details about someone, change names so that they can tell a version of the truth without fear of legal action. But Joe Lala is dead, which is an exceptionally good thing because it frees me to tell the real truth about him. You can't defame the dead, though nothing I'm going to say is defamatory anyway. Unfortunately, it's all true.

So yeah, I'm going to say his name: Joe Lala.

He died of lung cancer, and boy, I hope it hurt. And I've never felt like that about anyone. I am not someone who gains joy from others' pain; I've had enough pain in my own life to pray that no one else feels what I feel. By the time I was fifteen, I was telling my diary, *"Shit, if anyone read this, they'd think that my life was pretty bad…Druggy, alchi, violent stepfather doesn't sound like a nice life…"* I wouldn't wish this kind of feeling on anyone, so for me to be so virulent about Lala's death…and yet I make no apologies.

Lala was my "stepfather" from the time I was three years old until I was seven. When he died many years later there were gushing tributes to him — things like "To play with so many legends, you have to be a legend" — but the truth is, he was an abusive alcoholic and a junkie. He even burned my cereal spoons while shooting his heroin, but that wasn't close to the worst of it.

When my mother got with Lala, she was already having trouble sleeping—she had been through so much anxiety and pain after my dad left, and she was struggling. Misery loves company, and Lala told her he had this "herb" called China White that would help her get some rest. Nancy Priddy was from a place as close to true, innocent America as you can imagine: South Bend, Indiana, a safe, uncomplicated town where the worst people did was drink too much. And even though by the time she reached her twenties she had lived for a few years in very different places—the artistic, stoned streets of Laurel Canyon, California, and before that, the folk-filled streets of Greenwich Village, in New York—my mother didn't know drugs. This was so not the world she was from; she was dangerously naive about it. Given that she was desperate to get some rest, and that she trusted this new man in her life, she happily tried this herb called China White, and she slept. She felt great, so she took some more China White, she slept some more, on and on and on, all the way down the waterslide that is heroin addiction.

Being an addict like Lala was one thing; inveigling someone else into that world is another level of evil, especially someone as lost as my mother was in those years after my father left. The palpable selfishness, and the disregard for someone else's safety and health, shows me just what a terrible partner Joe Lala was to my mother. He'd found a weak, battered heart, and he had preyed upon it. He desperately needed someone next to him while he spiraled. It wouldn't have been any fun spiraling alone, so he brought my mother along for the terrible ride.

My mother always did the very best she could for me. But we suffered the twin scourges of poverty and trauma. We had both been left by a loved one; we were each a mirror to the pain the other was feeling.

What transpired was a childhood that, though it didn't involve malnutrition, as I would later learn my father's had, still had its fair share of deprivations. At home there were times when I'd think, *What's this fun powder in this baggie? Is it flour?* My mom would sometimes send me to school with tuna fish sandwiches in plastic bags, where they'd sit for hours in the California heat until lunchtime came around. We all could have died. In fact, I'm amazed more of us didn't die in the seventies.

There was no spare money for things even as cheap as hamburger buns, so we'd have hamburgers on white bread that would turn pink from the ketchup. I still remember the day she bought hamburger buns for the first time.

"Mom!" I said. "Thank you!"

I couldn't believe it. We were so rich. We had hamburger buns.

My mother managed to keep the truth of her addiction away from me, at least. You would never have known she was in such distress. She didn't behave any differently. I still loved lying in her lap, and she still smelled of that rose perfume.

I felt safe; I felt safe with her always. I always felt safe with my mommy...

I have incredible empathy for my mother.

She is my hero. She raised me alone; she would go on to survive cancer three times. But Joe Lala ruined my mom, putting her on a trajectory in which she would struggle with drug and alcohol abuse until only a decade or so ago.

The memories are burned into the backs of my retinas like sunlight. I sometimes think sharing the memories will lessen their power, but that's not the case. What Lala did, and who he was—and at such an important, formative time in my young life—compromised so many things a child needs: stability, tenderness, peace. Love. The safety supplied by my beautiful mother was critically challenged by the presence of this man who moved into our lives and brought with him a universe of hurt and danger.

It's difficult to even share some of the things he did. Like the day we came home to find Lala in a full drug nod, a bite of his own tuna sandwich in his mouth, a menthol cigarette still burning in his fingers, the ash at least an inch long. He could so easily have burned down the house and everyone in it. I can still see him now: he was in our garage room, wearing a short terry cloth robe, so stupidly short that you could almost see his balls.

Everything about him was disgusting, and frightening, and left me in a kind of emotional quicksand.

My mom always said, "I never met a junkie I didn't like because they tend to be lovely people." That's because they feel so damn good all the time, I guess. But Lala mixed his alcohol with the junk, which made him abusive and horrible.

Menthol and tuna and booze.

Mom had no income, no support, her family three thousand miles away, her ex-husband six hours north and in a new relationship. Being so alone, she sometimes left me in the "care" of a bunch of girls who lived in the Canyon.

"Care" is in quotation marks because they were all having sex with rock stars and didn't care about a little kid in the slightest.

Their wildness wasn't confined to their own exploits with adults either. In a world where there were no guardrails, it didn't matter to some of them what damage they did.

This is where the story darkens almost to black, and though I wish I could draw a veil across these pages, I also owe a debt of witness to that little girl who lived at 8723 Lookout Mountain Avenue, the house you could reach from both Lookout and Crescent Drive. But either way you found me, there I was, left to the whims of girls who were already promiscuous and unmoored from basic levels of morality and appropriate behavior.

Because. One day. One of the older ones. Well, she forced me. She made me.

I don't want to say it.

Fuck this.

She made me eat her out.

I was five years old.

I knew every part of it was wrong. I felt sick and scared and sad.

I owe that abused five-year-old this witness. It's not as if the adult I've become can effectively disassociate from what that girl went through either. It's not so much ripples on a pond as a great tsunami through life, the abuse leaving me in the thrall of shame when it comes to my sexuality. And it wasn't just my sexuality that was shattered; I have spent a lifetime with such incredibly low self-esteem I have put up with repeated ill use by partners and others.

But no, I never fully felt comfortable being touched, and that's true still. I have never felt comfortable with it my whole life, really, and all because of that girl forcing me to do something I barely understood but that I knew was shameful. This is how abuse works: the shame should have been hers, and lord knows, perhaps it is to this day. But it's damn sure mine. I already lived in a world where my safety was jeopardized every single day. I never knew if Lala was going to burn the house down, or beat one of us, and now the safety of being looked after by girls in the neighborhood was entirely compromised by this heinous, ruinous act forced upon me. Hurt people hurt people.

Damn a world in which a five-year-old girl is subjected to this kind of degradation. How I wish I never had to give words to what happened to her, but she is owed that at least.

In looking over my life, I'm reminded of a recent study suggesting a link between childhood trauma and an increased chance of developing MS. The 2022 study of eighty thousand Norwegian women, published in the *Journal of Neurology, Neurosurgery & Psychiatry,* noted three kinds of abuse of children that were possible factors in a subsequent diagnosis of the disease: sexual, emotional, and physical. Close to 20 percent of the women admitted to suffering one such form of abuse as a child (which is in and of itself a terrible number), but staggeringly, there was a 93 percent risk of an MS diagnosis if a child had been exposed to *all three*. And it's here your devastated narrator slowly raises her hand to sadly admit to all three, and then some.

My mind reels at this. To understand that the very things I survived could possibly chase me down and ravage my body with MS leaves me breathless with rage. I have fought my entire life to create peace for myself in the face of what happened to me as a child, only for that survival instinct to be rendered moot by damage to my telomeres.

It wasn't long after he moved in with us that the physical abuse of my mother by Lala started.

When I was about five, Lala punched and kicked my mother in a fierce assault, one borne of evil and drugs. It started with one of their usual fights but quickly escalated when my mom kicked him. At this, his rage coalesced into a closed-fist punch to the head, as hard as I'd ever seen anybody punch anybody.

She was knocked out.

I heard the scream of a little girl. "Don't do that to my mama!" It was me screaming, raising from my soul a sound as close to a banshee as I could manage with my tiny voice, from out of my tiny body.

"I hate you," I screamed at Lala. With this, he grabbed me by the back of my hair, lifted me up, and carried me to my bedroom—me screaming all the way—where he hurled me across the room and into the wall.

"You stay in here," he said. "You have nothing to do with this."

That was the little girl found by her godmother, Leanne, a little while later; Lala had fled. Leanne was one of the girls on the street who looked after me, though she was a good one. Sensing, perhaps, that something was amiss, or sent there by forces I'll never understand, Leanne had showed up and found me dazed by that wall, my mother beaten unconscious, sprawled out on our couch.

My mom would be out for the next day and well into the next night. I placed myself firmly at my mother's feet, hoping, I guess, to be a barrier to any further violence.

I would not be moved. I didn't care what anyone said: I wasn't leaving my mother's side.

"Christina," Leanne said to me at some point, "you have to go to bed." Night had already slipped up through the Canyon, the streetlights casting an odd glow across the room, as though this was the most peaceful scene imaginable, rather than a place of violence.

I kept my gaze fixed on my comatose mother.

"I'm not going to bed," I said to Leanne without looking at her.

I had a little purple tumbler that I'd stolen from my grandmother back in South Bend. I loved that thing;

I kept my toothbrush in it. Leanne, recognizing that there was no way I was moving anytime soon, kindly went and found it, and put some water in it for me. I just sat there, next to my unconscious mother, brushing my teeth over and over again, trying to clean away the stain of my five-year-old life, just waiting for her to wake up, waiting, waiting, brushing, waiting, the only sound in the room the dull clink of the toothbrush as I dipped it in the water over and over and over and over.

The fights between my mother and Joe Lala were terrible and violent, and I witnessed many of them. He would beat the shit out of her and then later, when the dust had settled, he'd say, "I love you so much, I was just drunk...," and she'd accept his excuses—I won't call them apologies—and on they would go.

But it wasn't just the fighting. A whole bunch of circus freaks came by all the time to score and do drugs. I would watch all these kooky weirdos and my mom snort heroin in the house. I even had a babysitter who stole cash from me because even though I was just a little girl, I was making a lot of money doing radio ads.

I first got my SAG card in 1975, on the back of a series of Kmart radio ads I'd done before I'd even turned five.

I often went with my mom on auditions, and in the case of the Kmart ads, she had a couple of friends who had been contracted to create them. One of them was the father of Josh Richman, who was making radio commercials at the time, and as I was young and had a cute little voice, they would use me, too.

Kmart was one of the first major stores to process photographic film in bulk for regular consumers, and as part of the promotion for this newfangled service, they promised to refund amateur photographers if their pictures were bad. This promise—"goof-proof"—was to be advertised via the sweet, cherubic voices of Josh Richman, playing Jeffry, and a little young me, playing Chrissie. We were the goof-proof kids, and those ads ran for years. We even won a Clio advertising award during their run, and I earned enough from being cute and goof-proof that my mother could invest my income in property in the Canyon.

In one of the ads, Josh says, "When I say 'Action!,' you say, 'You get a goof-proof guarantee on picture processing at Kmart.'"

"I can't say all that," I reply. "My mouth is too little." And though it was a cute line, it was also true: the producers had to splice together consonants and vowels to make my toddler burble sound like actual, comprehensible English. But it worked, and suddenly I had a SAG card.

By the time I turned seven, I was earning real

money for my mom and me—in fact, I have never stopped working since that time, at least until I got MS. I did ads for cat chow and canned ham, and then I started doing episodics, including classics like *Family Ties* and *Charles in Charge*. (It was in those days that I met dear, much-mourned Matthew Perry.) When I wasn't working or in school, I was in acting classes, and I still tell people to never stop training because you're never going to be as good as you think you are, a lesson I learned early and often.

From a very young age, working was my identity, my everything. Being on set was where I felt most comfortable. I had to be someone I wasn't, and I found that in the guise of a character I could protect the little scared me. When I was working, I had to be on time and respectful and professional. That world was organized and had rules. I got to escape into someone I wasn't.

From the start, working was survival. I was pretty much always the sole breadwinner at home. That's been a bone of contention my whole life. I love my mom; she would do little acting things here and there or get the lead in a commercial, but the truth was, I was making all the money. It was hard for her—my dad never paid child support, meaning there were times when we were on food stamps, and other times when we had nothing at all. So working was never a conscious decision I made; it was how we survived. I got good at it because I had to do it. I had no choice.

That working kid bought a house, a place we rented out until I moved into it when I was seventeen.

But that fledgling actor was still very afraid of Lala. I hated him so much, yet at the same time, I knew we were dependent on him. He had a lot of money, he bought me things, he cared for us financially to make up for his lack of care physically and emotionally. But he managed to turn my mom into a weak, pathetic human being, so deep down I still hated him. After Lala, my mother was never the same.

Sometimes if my mom and I got into a fight—the usual mother-daughter stuff—she would leave the house, and I'd be alone for hours, screaming and screaming and screaming because I wasn't sure she was ever coming back.

Those are just some of the visions that fill my head when I'm stuck on my bed in my house in Laurel Canyon, just a mile as the raven flies from that house on Lookout Mountain Avenue. MS makes the simplest tasks excruciating, nauseating, tiring…I'm so often beyond tired. Sure, I have a large house way up on the mountain now, but some days I'm back there in our

750-square-foot house, the row house you could reach from two different streets.

Someone asked me recently about *comfort:* What do I do for comfort, what comforts me the most in my new life of disability and painful stasis? I knew straightaway what my answer would be: "Nag champa, chimes, and a fire in the fireplace." This has been a mantra for me since I was very little. These are the things—along with the horrors and my mother's comatose body and that tumbler from South Bend—that I brought with me from my childhood, things that on a good day almost outweigh the Joe Lalas and the "caregivers" and the abuse and the addicted mothers of Laurel Canyon. My mother always burned nag champa, and there were always chimes tinkling in the windows, and we never wanted for a fire. In my journal from November 1988, I wrote, *"Momma had a nervous breakdown this morning. So I bought her a TV and built a fire and put out candles and shit. I spent the rest of the evening with her. It was really nice. I think she had a good time."*

We return to the primal things whenever we need solace. For others it might be a song like "For What It's Worth (Stop, Hey What's That Sound)," or a photo album filled with pressed flowers, or a car like a Nova heaving down a hill. For me it's the holy trinity of Laurel Canyon: nag champa, chimes, and a fire in the fireplace.

You with the Sad Eyes

* * *

Lala finally left us when I was seven. He grew convinced that my mom was crazy, and he had been calling my dad to say that my mother was an unfit parent, which was incredible given how terrible Lala had been to her. By then my mother had almost physically disappeared, and great, unfathomable damage had been done to both of us.

One day my father came to one of my school recitals and told me he was taking me for pizza. I protested that I needed to tell my mom, who was in the bathroom, but he said it wasn't an issue, and stole me away, putting me in the back of the car and driving me back to his house in Woodland Hills.

When my mom came out of the bathroom and realized I was gone, she was, not surprisingly, completely hysterical. Fortunately, she was able to quickly figure out who'd taken me—I presume someone saw what had happened and told her—and she rushed to Woodland Hills to confront my father. I am told there was a terrible scene when she arrived—windows were broken, hair pulled out of heads, screaming and shouting, things said that could never be taken back…

Now, when I corral my mind to think of those days, there is sometimes a blank where disaster once was.

This has nothing to do with the multiple lesions on my brain from MS. Instead, I think at some point my memory short-circuited, given the out-of-control drama of my young life. I do remember being mad at my mom, though, but I was mad at my father, too. I think I was mad at everyone; I'm not sure anyone could have blamed me for that.

Through it all my mother had tried to keep me innocent of the vagaries of the adults around me, but children, even if they don't know the details, can easily and instinctually sense the tenor of a room, and I know that little girl understood all too well that the world was a dangerous, unforgiving place. Yes, there was nag champa and my mother's rose perfume, but there was also the stench of violence, of loss, of being pulled this way and that by two people who couldn't work out how to raise me together.

After the terrible events in Woodland Hills, my mom, leaving me with my dad, decamped somewhere out of town, where she tried to kill herself. She seemed to think that with my father taking me to Woodland Hills, she'd never get to see me again, and that was too much to bear. She had to get her stomach pumped after a dangerous overdose. I can't remember how long she was gone. Again, my memory short-circuits. I don't suppose it was longer than two weeks, but to me back then, it was an eternity. I remember my child mind fixating on how I didn't even have any clothes with me, as it had all happened so suddenly.

Then I remember her pulling up to my dad's house in the blue Nova, alive, a returning angel, and I couldn't wait to get in the car with her.

She was my sanctuary. My mother was home. And that's where we headed, the two of us silent on the 101, my heart leaping at the sight of the communications tower above the Mulholland Tennis Club, a beacon of returning, bright and sharp above Laurel Canyon.

Looking back, perhaps the most important thing I take away from that photograph these days is my smile—I am happy. I'm with my beloved grandparents, and though Lala and my mother, sadly, are probably both as high as kites on heroin at the time, she loved me and I knew she loved me and I felt safe with her, always.

THREE

THE BATHROOM FLOOR

MANY YEARS LATER, WHEN my mother discovered that Lala had cancer, she called him to see how he was.

When I asked her why she'd done such a thing, she said, "Well, I have to find *closure*."

"Closure to what, Mom?" I said. "Closure for ruining your daughter's life, for ruining *your* life, for destroying anything I could have had at the most formative time, taking that away from me and leading me toward a lifetime of attracting abusive junkie dicks to my life?"

Despite my anger, deep down I partly understand why she made that call, though it hurts to think she did so. We are all bound to create patterns we can barely break. And the bad people around us bring their patterns, too, which we fold into because we're more comfortable with the pain we know than the threat of the unknown. Bad people like Lala cause damage, and then they apologize; they vilify, and then they smooth-talk; they create huge mounds of shit, and make the shit seem like it's your fault.

As for my mother, well, she'd been so financially dependent on that man, trying to raise a child with scant income and few job prospects, that she'd put up with so much more than she should have because there were mouths to feed.

So yes, all those years later she called him. She was bound upon her wheel, trapped inside her patterns, and was still hostage to him, too, I guess. I don't know what she expected to hear, what kinds of words he could put together for her to feel closure. That's for her to understand; her daughter, though, had a suspicion that all the greatest words imaginable could never make up for twenty-four hours of brushing her teeth, waiting for her mother to wake up and make it better.

Abuse doesn't happen just once. And it doesn't just affect one person. The model, this great pattern of hurt, had been created, the journey set before I'd even had the chance to understand I was on a journey in the first place. I was growing up the daughter of a mother trapped in a traumatic, abuse-ridden house, and I was to have that model as my very own for much of the rest of my life, too.

Now all I had to do was live it.

* * *

Back in L.A., reunited with her daughter but deeply alone again, my mother somehow kicked heroin on our bathroom floor all by herself (I was staying with my father during her detox). This was a truly heroic deed; I can't imagine how she did it, not for a second. She later told me that it was the worst thing she'd ever dealt with in her entire life, but she'd done it so that she would never have to face being away from me again. She had to be there for me forever, so she fought back against the drugs and got clean.

She said that as she detoxed alone, she had wanted to rip the skin off of those fragile bones because of the pain. With heroin withdrawal, the body aches, you get palpitations, anxiety, insomnia, chills, diarrhea. You vomit, you scream with tears, you get feverish, you sweat. It's a brutal, unforgiving detox, perhaps the worst detox a person can go through.

And my mother did it alone on the bathroom floor.

She is my hero. Our relationship, though sometimes fraught, has long settled into one of love and acceptance, but even back then, she taught me what it means to survive something terrible and emerge into a kind of bliss, akin to freedom. Sometimes an anger swells in me when I think of what we went through, what Lala put her through, and yes, what my father did to her by leaving us both right at the start of my life. But more and more that anger is replaced by gratitude, by acceptance, by understanding what she was able to build out of the chaos. I know now just how strong she had to be for both of us. I finally understand what it takes to put your own needs to one side because you love someone so much that all you can think about is their happiness. It took becoming a mother myself to fully comprehend just what my own mother achieved.

I'll never stop thinking about her life back then: imagine the strength it took to quit heroin cold turkey on a bathroom floor. Imagine having no support to help raise your kid. Imagine wanting love but knowing that you have to put your kid first. Imagine the fear she must have felt in trusting anyone, let alone a man, after what Lala put us through.

When I was growing up, it was always just the two of us, so if it was often lonely and traumatic for me, imagine how hard it was for her. As I've grown older, I've been more able to find the heroism in my mother, the selflessness. And I'm grateful for that.

And there was joy, too.

We used to drive up the 5 freeway to Magic Mountain all the time, just the two of us, and always on Mother's Day. I can't imagine that many mothers would choose a trip to Magic Mountain for their special day, but she knew how much I loved it, so it became a family tradition, me hoping each year that I was finally tall enough to be allowed on the Gold Rusher, the Log Jammer, the Colossus, or the Great American Revolution. And given what we'd both been through—the violence, the fear, the struggle to just survive—we'd think nothing of those huge roller coasters, whooping and hollering as our stomachs got left behind, free for a few minutes from the pressures of our shared pasts, our challenging presents, and our uncertain futures.

The two of us—always the two of us. Some weekends we'd drive down off the mountain and head to the coast. We'd roller-skate through Venice all the way up to Santa Monica, which at the time wasn't the safest thing to do, despite the lo-fi, retro filter through which we now view the seventies. It might have been the era of free love, but there was plenty of hatred, too—we'd see blood splatters on the bike trail that hugs the beach because some dudes in jean shorts had been fighting drunk again. But I was never afraid—my mom always made me feel safe, that I was okay, that no one would get me. We'd buy a hot dog on a stick, or a corn dog, or even a cheese corn dog if we were feeling fancy, and then on we'd roll until the sun started to set and the L.A. chill descended.

In the end, I became a really good skater, joined a troop, the whole bit. We were even highlighted in the opening shots of an episode of *CHiPs*, rolling along the boardwalk in Venice. It's funny to me how even my hobbies would end up as jobs; we were thankful, as ever, for the work.

Other weekends, when I wasn't with my dad in Woodland Hills, my mom and I would head south to Laguna Beach, where we'd stay at the Laguna Riviera, a beachfront motel with an indoor pool on the street side. There was no room service, just a Danish and a cup of coffee in a Styrofoam cup in the lobby. We'd eat at a cool little vegetarian stand around the corner, and that's how it was: just the two of us.

One such weekend my mom suddenly said, "Let's go to Tijuana!," just over the border into Mexico, about a hundred miles south of Laguna. We sang "Cuanto Le Gusta" all the way there, which was funny as we often didn't have a dime, but we had a happy time, just like the song says.

We'd long since given up the Nova and now my mom drove a sage-green used Cadillac, and I felt like I was in an episode of *Lifestyles of the Rich and Famous.* Once we'd crossed the border, we bought a pair of sombreros and a little purse for me that had, confusingly enough, ACAPULCO written on it.

I put all my money in that purse, but one of my junkie babysitters stole it. I still get mad when I think of it — $300, which was a lot in 1979.

* * *

Once my mom was off the heroin, it's hardly surprising that she turned to Valium to calm her nerves. She was, as they say, "California sober," meaning she'd quit the really bad stuff. She had bad anxiety and constantly fussed about her weight. Some of those issues surely rubbed off on me. Some years later, when I was probably twelve or thirteen, my mom sent me to school with a bottle of pills all my own. At first, it was a mixture of diet pills.

My mom always thought I could lose a little weight. She made me go to Weight Watchers, and we always had Weight Watchers food in the house for her. I was in my teens and no longer teeny tiny anymore. I had hips, and a butt, and my mom would often say, "You could stand to lose five pounds." But we were all a product of the times as much as anything. These were the days informed by ads like the one for the diet cola Tab, in which a honey-voiced male actor croons over a sickly song, "When you can't be with him, be in his mind. Be a 'mind sticker,' with a shape he can't forget."

This was standard stuff in the seventies zeitgeist, and my home was no different.

The issues of the time became her issues, and her issues became mine, and soon she started sending me to school with my own stash of Valium. Those she told me to chew so they activated faster. One day I got into a fight with some kid and chewed all the pills. When my mom came to pick me up, I was lying on the cot in the nurse's office. She was so mad she threw her keys at me.

"What the fuck is wrong with you?" she said.

Drugs were everywhere in the Canyon by that point, and the days of weed had long been supplanted by a darker scene.

One of the renters we took on to fill the garage was a weird guy named Alan Burke. Not only did he provide some much-needed income, but his presence also offered some additional babysitting for me.

My mom sometimes left me with Burke while she went to auditions or to the work that came from auditions, and one night I remember going into the garage to find a huge mirror on his bed and a ton of people around the mirror.

I had no idea what they were doing, but I knew it wasn't right. *Who are all these people? Why is there a mirror on the bed in the (illegal) garage apartment? And why are they so intently focusing on it like it contains the meaning of the universe?*

The people around the mirror didn't notice that there was a little kid—probably no more than five years old—just knocking about, watching them. Actually, they may have noticed and just not cared. They weren't even friends of Burke; they were there to try out whatever drugs he had that day before buying a baggie of whatever worked best for their fucked-up minds. Burke was like those middle-aged women in supermarkets forcing chips and the latest salsa on shoppers who were trying to just get their shopping done. Only in this case, I realize now that it wasn't salsa; it was cocaine and heroin and God knows what else.

There are times I'm still pissed about what I was exposed to as a kid. My mom and I have talked about it so many times, and I have to believe her when she says she just simply wasn't aware. She had so much else going on that it was hard for her to see what was in front of her.

All these years later, I can only assume that she knew Burke was a drug dealer, but I think the South Bend, Indiana, in her didn't want to believe such things. She'd been through so much that I think for a while it became impossible to fully comprehend where her life had taken her, and what difficult things it asked of her daughter.

My young heart felt the stress of it, the danger, the fact that it was transgressive, and that these people were strangers and were acting oddly, manically, urgently.

I stood there and I watched them. I knew I deserved better.

So much for Burke, my "babysitter." The best I can say is that a crowd of addicts around a mirror was at least a better situation than the party I was taken to a couple of doors down around that time. It was at some musician's house. I don't know why I went or who took me; those were still the days when the Canyon was a small community and everyone was invited to everything, doors were open, people came and went. But at some point during the party, the musician felt it was his right to run his hand up along my leg. I remember crying and him laughing at me. Everything after is black, once again the dark veil pulled hard across my memory, so I don't really know what happened.

These were the kinds of scary things that the adults were doing to little children in Laurel Canyon.

I think my mom sensed my discomfort, though she didn't know the full extent of what I'd been going through. She knew enough to start me on what has become a lifelong practice of meditation, weaving spirituality into my childhood. She taught me to think in metaphysical ways from an early age, which helped save my soul from the worst excesses of what was going on, even if my body was constantly put in places of danger and turmoil.

For a while my mother had been trying to find something in her life, something that might hold back the pain into which she had been thrust by Lala. In the late seventies, she'd read a book by Shakti Gawain called *Creative Visualization.* In that now-classic book, Gawain argues that we can create a better life for ourselves by changing our inner visions. My mother was taking what she'd learned and teaching me that I must be careful how I think and talk about myself—as she once said, there's no one more tortured than a metaphysician who's not practicing. So I learned to practice creative visualization, which to my mind is really just another form of prayer.

As a young girl I suffered greatly from anxiety and insomnia. I found myself unhinged by all the unanswered questions about the world around me. "If you fell off the face of the earth, you wouldn't land. But if you did land, then we're inside of something, which means there's a bottom to that something, but still, you wouldn't land." "This thing has a name, this thing has a reason, this thing has its place. We're in a car, we're in a house, we're in a country, but the universe is infinite?" "We're taught that everything has a beginning, a middle, and an end. But there's no end to grief? Grief just changes colors."

All these things and more would keep me up at night. My mom would get into bed with me and try to calm me down with her newfound practices of meditation and visualization. She'd say, "Imagine your forehead is a chalkboard—erase everything and write what you want to see instead." I know now that visualization is more about thinking our way into happiness and joy and health, giving to the universe so that the universe returns good things to us, et cetera, but as a little girl, rather than inviting karma—a concept altogether too advanced for my young soul—I would visualize walking down a beach while filming a TV show in which I was the star...just me and, oh, all five members of Duran Duran.

John Taylor, especially, was the Man. I was pretty sure I was going to marry him. He may not have known that yet, but that didn't stop me from imagining it as a real option for my future. To seal the deal, even though I was still a preteen, I would go to Duran Duran concerts and write stuff on T-shirts and put them into the bins they provided for fans to give things to the band. (That's what we all fervently believed; now, of course, I'm pretty sure the band never saw any of it.)

Because the universe has no timeline, many years later I starred on a sitcom about a woman with retrograde amnesia called *Samantha Who?*, and the script called for my character to have a rock star boyfriend. Someone on the show announced that they were friends with John Taylor of Duran Duran...and hey, presto, there I was as an adult person, and the love of my life, at least as a child, was opposite me, playing Tommy Wylder, my boyfriend on my show, a show that I had also visualized as a little girl.

As a ten-year-old, I was sure that John Taylor was

going to be my husband at some point. He wasn't, but don't let anyone tell you visualization doesn't work. For years I held in my head the vision of a punk rock God—I would always see him in my meditations. And then in 1994 he appeared. I was sitting at the Kibitz Room, next door to the famous Canter's Deli on Fairfax in Los Angeles. I was eating French fries with gravy (this vegetarian was naive enough to think gravy didn't have meat in it). A guy came around the corner, and my punk rock God manifestation snapped into view.

There he was, bleached blond hair, missing teeth, a brown button-down shirt over a T-shirt. Literally my breath was taken away. *It's my punk rock God,* I thought. *It's my punk rock fantasy.*

I'll get to that. But back in 1981, I was all about John Taylor, Duran Duran, and trying to survive the various demons of Laurel Canyon.

Despite the creeping darkness of the 1980s, I couldn't help but still feel the magic of Laurel Canyon. To this day, one of my favorite things is the smell of the Canyon after it rains. There's something so poignant to me about the aroma of damp leaves on the ground, the petrichor rich and pungent, the streets near the Wonderland school always slick with runoff, the night-blooming jasmine and eucalyptus filling my head with magic and hope. Each day as a kid, I'd walk up the hill of Lookout Mountain from Wonderland, which I attended until middle school, and I'd find my young self completely embracing this beautiful, magical fragrance. I was all by myself, autonomous, in a world where I desperately wanted safety and a star on the Boulevard. Then I'd reach our house, and a new perfume would envelop me, the nag champa and the fireplace, and as the chimes clanged at the windows, a powerful, otherworldly feeling of calm would come over me.

By this point, with Lala gone and my mother miraculously clean, I didn't want to leave; I'm still that way, a home person. I just want to stay by my hearth, because the world out there remains frightening to me. Even as a child if my friends wanted to hang out — Mariah, Miranda, Jody, Luke — I always had them come to my house. On the odd occasion when I'd go down to Mariah's house — she lived across the street from the school — on the way down the hill I would do jetés in the middle of the street so that I could get there faster.

One day a girl named Pharel strode up to me in Laurel Canyon and asked me for a cigarette. We've been friends ever since. Early in our friendship we were in her room, where she and her friends liked to smoke pot. I tried it; we had gotten a pizza from a place called Two Guys from Italy and couldn't stop cracking up. I'll never forget Pharel saying, "I haven't laughed this hard from being high since I was a kid." She was only thirteen years old.

We all shared the sense of the music of this canyon and the lore of the Canyon and the feeling of what it had been, but we also felt something scary there, too. Behind our closed doors, bad things were happening, and to all of us. We were all only children with single parents, single moms. Many of the guys who came into our mothers' lives were bad, bad men. They were the embodiment of the poor judgment of our desperate, sad mothers, who had had a dream of a family taken from them, only to replace it with distracted decisions, or relationships that started in rainbows and ended in fire.

Consequently, our childhoods veered toward the dark. None of us had yards to play in, and few of us had siblings, so we'd fill our time trying to steal our moms' pot or booze. Then there was the day my friend Lucy got mad at my friend Heather and chased her a full mile up the hill with a butcher's knife. Heather, desperately needing protection, headed for my house, burst in, and cowered in my kitchen. Seeing the huge knife, followed by Lucy, coming around the corner, I pulled a six-pack of Diet Coke out of the fridge and hurled it at Lucy's head to make her stop. This did indeed end the confrontation, only for both of them to turn on me.

"You're so *emotional,* Christina," Heather said.

You with the Sad Eyes

* * *

I don't suppose it helped that I really didn't want Nancy Priddy to be with anyone else after Joe Lala. I was so afraid of who that man might be, and the shit he'd bring into our lives, that I probably suffocated her in some ways, but I just didn't want anyone else to hurt her.

Well into the 1980s my mom was still involved in the music scene—whenever we went to New York, for example, she'd see her former producer, Phil Ramone. By then he'd produced everyone—the Simon twins, Carly and Paul; Celine Dion and Dionne Warwick; Pavarotti; my dear friend growing up Mark Volman, of the band the Turtles; and Peter, Paul, and Mary—and when my mom still hung around with him, he was working with Billy Joel. For a while my mother had a relationship with one of the members of Billy's band. We went to stay at the guy's place on Long Island for a couple of months, but I was very much in my "Keep Mom single" phase, so one day I jumped up on his bed and pissed all over it.

It seems I was eventually forgiven because Billy Joel himself made me my first banana and peanut butter sandwich. We were in his kitchen with his whole family, and I can still see him peeling a banana, slicing it right down the middle, and filling it with peanut butter. Long Island clearly wasn't the land of warm tuna sandwiches — Billy's PB & banana was, up to that point in my life, the single best thing I'd ever eaten.

We spent a lot of time on the East Coast because we had family there and because my mother is a New Yorker at heart. She'd take me to every single Broadway show back then (there was no age limit in the eighties). I was tiny when I saw *A Chorus Line* for the first time, featuring the legendary original cast — Donna McKechnie, Kelly Bishop, Priscilla Lopez, Robert LuPone, and Wayne Cilento, who'd choreograph *Sweet Charity* years later on Broadway — and I also had the pleasure of seeing *The Wiz* and *Ain't Misbehavin'*. It all just blew my mind. The bug to perform, especially the song-and-dance bug, was birthed in me during those visits.

My mom had put me in dance classes at three years old, another trick she thought would keep me sane, along with meditation. Dance immediately became central to my life. From the age of three, I've done ballet, tap, jazz, modern, Fosse... everything. Even if I didn't feel good, or if I didn't want to, or was angry or scared or anxious or heartbroken, my mother would always say, "This is nonnegotiable. You're going to dance class."

Having escaped her own addictions, my mom wanted me to have a positive addiction, which was to dance, wanted me to have somewhere I could go to express myself, something positive to become obsessed with. Dance became the thing that saved me, and has saved me ever since. Dance, even more than acting, was my whole life. Not being able to dance as I once did now that I have MS is one of the hardest things about the disease. It's impossible to overstate how important dance is to me. Not just as an expression of my artistic nature, but as a kind of therapy that goes beyond talking, beyond "closure," beyond making peace with the past. I love dance more than anything in life. It calms me, inspires me, moves me, brings me fully into my body, expresses all the hurt and anger and sorrow I've felt across the years. For most of my adult life, I've had a dance studio in my house, no matter where I am, replete with the suspension floors, barres, everything. Even the house I funded at seven years old, on Love Street behind the Laurel Canyon Country Store, had one. There was a tiny downstairs apartment that came with that property, and much later I made that whole thing a dance studio. (That downstairs section had formerly been where everyone in the Canyon went to cultivate their pot.) I would go down there for hours, just by myself, dancing out my past, dancing into what I hoped would be a happier future.

These days, I prop myself up on pillows, my cats and dog ranged around me like sentries, and I watch old Bob Fosse dances on a loop. There he is now, slithering across the desert performing his snake dance in the 1974 movie *The Little Prince,* inventing moves that would be copied count for count by Michael Jackson a decade later. There's *Fosse's* moonwalk, there's *Fosse's* spinning of the trilby, *Fosse's* leg pops, *Fosse's* spats on his black shoes, and yes, *Fosse's* crotch grab.

Occasionally, I'll still dance. I sent a video to a friend recently of me dancing to R.E.M.'s "Everybody Hurts." As Michael Stipe sings, a couple of times I regain my balance holding on to a credenza, but otherwise I'm out there on my own, dancing my ass off. I still have the angles, the reach, the positions as natural as breathing. Late in the song I find a huge smile breaking across my face as all thoughts of MS recede and I'm just dancing, dancing as though I'm perfectly healthy, as though I have not been through cancer and MS and loss and trauma. Because that's what dance gives me: a place where joy and love win all the battles against darkness and fear.

But then I tire, and the pain returns, and it's as if the music itself retreats, until all I can hear are the chimes at my window, ringing as if to call the ghosts back to life.

My mother and I also regularly went east to Indiana to visit family.

My maternal grandmother, Katherine Iona Driggs,

was one of the most incredible human beings I've ever met in my life; she was everything to me. It's so poignant, the things we remember of a person we loved. For me it was that she didn't have a coffee maker, so she always drank Folgers instant coffee, and if you wanted a cup, you were pointed to the Folgers crystals and a kettle. To this day that particular taste takes me right back to those moments of my life.

Katherine was a tiny woman with a little puff at her belly—I used to call her Jelly Roll because she felt squishy. We went to South Bend every Christmas to see her, to her perfect Victorian home on Victoria Street with its gently pitched roof. It was just Mom and me; we always slept in my mom and her sister's room, in their twin beds from when they were kids. There was a smell to the house that I can still remember—something Midwestern and I guess Folgers-y that comforted me throughout all those challenging years of my childhood.

I remember every winter being freezing cold. I was a Laurel Canyon kid, but hell, the Indiana snow was up to our knees so I think anyone would have felt it.

My grandma smelled like the perfume Charlie. Years later, after she died, I took a bottle of it from her house and sometimes I'll just put it on to remember her while I sip a Folgers. Every Christmas my uncle Tommy and his family would come from Naperville, Illinois, and we'd eat from the same menu for Thanksgiving and Christmas. The stuffing was filled with raisins, water chestnuts, onion, celery...no sage — that's too fancy. (Actually, my grandma had to make two different stuffings each year: one for us, and one for my uncle Tom, who required an oyster dressing. As a kid I never understood what that even meant except that I guessed it had oysters in it? Ew.) We'd have green bean casserole with Campbell's cream of mushroom soup, spiced up with a little bit of soy sauce — one of the recipes from the side of the can. Basic super salty mashed potatoes. My mom would always make creamed corn, too, with crumbled-up, buttered saltines on top. There were biscuits, also from a can.

No salad.

Being in Indiana brought me such a beautiful feeling of family that I didn't otherwise have. I was the very first grandchild, and I'm not sure what my grandma knew about what was going on in my mom's life; either way, she turned a blind eye to a lot of it. I don't think my mom shared too much either.

Most days we'd go up to the top of Victoria Hill and sled down. I remember that at the bottom of the hill we'd be racing toward Route 31, which to a small kid seemed like a roaring freeway. If you didn't stop before you reached it, you ran the risk of ending up like Frogger — that is, very dead. But we'd sled that hill over and over and over, until our lungs ached from the cold and our fingers could no longer hold the rope.

Other days we'd go cross-country skiing out west of the city, in Bendix Woods County Park.

Back at my grandmother's house, sometimes when the family got too loud, I'd head down to her basement to get away from everybody upstairs. It was a magical room with a pool table half the usual size. The basement walls were decorated with art. My grandfather, who died before I was born, had been a musician and an artist and a photographer. When he was alive, he would take beautiful black-and-white portraits of people and then paint over them — essentially, colorizing them by hand — and hang them on those walls.

There were no addictions in South Bend, no mean people. At least not until I was much older. No one was creepy. We'd all wear Christmas sweaters; there would be game shows on the TV. I'd wake up in the morning and find my grandmother watching General Hospital, sipping on her Folgers.

I would think, "This is what other people do."

Meanwhile, the Canyon kept slipping in the other direction.

One night when I was nine years old, we were awakened by the constant whir of helicopter blades. Helicopters are an integral part of Los Angeles life — the LAPD helicopter squad is the biggest in the country, and local TV stations use them to cover news and car chases—so we didn't immediately think too much of it. But when they didn't stop all night, we knew something bad had happened.

Less than a mile away, at 8763 Wonderland Avenue, the cops had found a scene of unimaginable horror. Neighbors had heard screaming but either figured it was just someone doing gestalt therapy—it was Laurel Canyon, after all—or were so used to noise from the house that they hadn't thought to call the police until much later. The headline of an Associated Press article published two days later, on July 3, 1981, read SCREAMS OF VICTIMS DIDN'T ALERT NEIGHBORS and went on to say, "Four people killed in a house where screams were so commonplace that neighbors ceased to notice were beaten in a struggle... Several neighbors said they had heard screams, moans, and cries of 'Please don't kill me!' in the early morning hours Wednesday, but had paid no attention."

When the police finally did arrive, they found four people who had been pulverized to death: Barbara Richardson, Ron Launius, Joy Miller, and William "Billy" Deverell had all been murdered by beatings. Launius, Miller, and her boyfriend, Deverell, had been members of a cocaine-dealing group, the Wonderland Gang, and the house itself was a known drug-dealing spot.

A few weeks earlier, various members of the Wonderland Gang had robbed an underworld character called Eddie Nash, the sleazy owner of the Kit Kat Club strip club; they stole drugs, cash, heroin, jewelry, and even antique guns from the mobster. The gang had made it into Nash's house thanks to John Holmes, an infamous porn star. Holmes had visited his pal Nash to score drugs and had then left a side door purposefully unlocked so that his friends in the gang could easily gain entry.

It's widely believed that the murders of July 1, 1981 — known now as the Wonderland Murders — were part of a payback scheme for the Nash heist. The murders are to this day unsolved, but they were horribly brutal: each of the deceased was bludgeoned to death, which must be one of the very worst ways to die. Only one person who was present that night survived: Ron Launius's wife, Susan. Her terrible injuries left her with amnesia and brain damage, and she was therefore unable to help the detectives. The only reason she survived was because after she was bludgeoned, she fell off the bed and against a wall, which served to keep her brains inside her skull.

I was not yet ten years old when the Wonderland murders happened, but I developed a kind of sick fascination with what had taken place just around the corner from where I lived. When someone came over, we'd say, "Do you want to go see the murder house?," and my mom and I would take people up the street to go look at the bloody mattresses left discarded in the carport. I vividly remember all the windows having some kind of white substance on them — I'd later learn it was the stuff they use to get blood off. The house itself was still blocked off with police tape, but TV cameras remained a constant, as did my mother and I, driving by to show friends where all this dreadful slaughter had happened.

I was mostly numb to the violence. A friend's mom had been shot to death by her boyfriend in the neighborhood, and we never even talked about it. There was crazy shit happening all around us. By the time the Wonderland murders took place, it felt more like a movie than real life, and because it didn't feel real, it couldn't truly hurt me. Instead, it was exciting. It never fully registered as horrifying until I grew up and looked back on it all.

It turns out that the Wonderland murders were a watershed; things started to improve in the following months and years. Jerry Brown, then the governor of California, had a house around the corner from the murders in the Canyon, and with his influence, things got safer. But the Wonderland murders were such a symbol of how far the Canyon had come from the days of wampum beads and two cats in the yard. Coke was rampant; the shadowy bends of the narrow streets seemed more sinister than ever. What had happened to my mother, and me, behind closed doors in recent years seemed to be echoed in the dark turn this once beautiful place had suffered.

Many years later, I heard that there was a movie being made about the Wonderland murders, and I met with the director, James Cox, at the Chateau Marmont to talk about the project. I felt a deep need to be part of the movie.

"I don't know how I'm going to get into this movie, but I have to. The people who understood that night were Canyonites. You're not going to find anyone who actually lived through that like I did," I told him. "I don't care who I play; in fact, I'll play John Holmes's penis if that's what it takes." (At five foot five I figured I was roughly the same size as the porn star's infamous dick.)

Cox said, "Do you want to play Susan Launius?" — that is, the only survivor. It immediately felt right. I knew everything about Susan. I knew what happened to her. I knew intimate details of the crime scene. I knew it all. I was the only person involved in the movie who had actually been there, not in the house but in the canyon. I would have played anyone in that movie, but to be given the role of Susan felt like divine alignment.

As preparation for the role, I made a visit to 8763 Wonderland Avenue to get a sense of it, although given my obsession with it, I already knew every room where the murders and assaults had taken place. (I was also the *young child* who read *Helter Skelter,* the book about the Manson murders, so often that I can still quote great chunks of it verbatim.) As I walked around 8763, I could still feel the violence, the horror palpable, the air sticky with blood and bludgeoning. It was as if the walls held the unanswered screams. There was the very wall where Susan Launius's brain matter was staunched, and there was the spot where Joy Miller was found on her bed...At the time, a bunch of young dudes lived at 8763—rockabillies who rode Triumphs—and I was eager to find out if they too felt anything, felt the horror and mayhem, the dark, sinister echoes of a once-terrible time.

They said they didn't feel a thing.

But I did. Sometimes I still do.

FOUR

QUIT

"I did another episode of *Charles in Charge* this week. It was great. I get the best feeling when I'm on that lot."
From my diary, January 12, 1985

THINGS IMPROVED ALL OVER the Canyon after Wonderland. Except in my brain, that is.

My mom has said that when I hit my teens, she loathed me, the only time in my life that she actively hated my guts. I was so depressed, and such a horrible little asshole because of it. I can hardly blame her.

Whenever I sneak into my secret metal box and read my diary from those years, an image crystallizes of a sad, innocent, complicated kid. I find that at age twelve, I've described myself as "5' 5", 110 pounds, white blonde with green eyes." Under "In Case of

Emergency Please Notify," I've written, "Please let me die!," although at some point later I had scribbled out that particular plea. There's my home address, and there, under "Business Address," I've written "20th Cen Fox."

Amidst all the usual teen angst about friendships and love there are the first signs that I'm incredibly hard on myself, especially when it comes to my physical appearance. In 1984, I write in regard to a guy named Mike, "I wish he would like me, but I'm too ugly." Ten days later I tell my diary, "You won't believe who I'm going out with... Mike." I read these pages now and can see how my mind was catastrophizing. My fling with Mike doesn't save me from my inner critic, though.

I was hell on my mom in those days. By early 1985, I'm writing, "I love my mom very much, we just haven't been getting along very well." As my teen years went on, it was as if my mind became like a witch's mind, fighting against me half the time. My mom caught me smoking in front of the teenage dance club, Hot Trax, on Van Nuys Boulevard. It wasn't just the two of us against the world anymore. I was sneaking out and rebelling. I got in so much trouble.

I was desperate to be that "normal" rebellious high schooler from all those John Hughes movies, although in my case my hair was shaved on both sides, and I was wearing combat boots, fishnets, and a pillowcase for a skirt. Instead I was always working. Even though I wouldn't admit it at the time, I think it was work that ultimately got me through.

I don't know what would've happened to me without work. Given the world I grew up in, I'm guessing that, for a start, I was a candidate for some serious addiction issues, although my mom always said to me, "If you ever do drugs, I will kill you and I'll kill whoever gave them to you."

But working saved me because I had one clear thing to do: I had to show up on a set, be an adult, and nail the scene. I never look back and wish I'd had a different life, at least in regard to working from such a young age.

Though maybe once...

When I was thirteen — probably only a few weeks after that diary entry above about how much I loved *Charles in Charge* — I told my mom I was quitting acting.

"I don't want to do this anymore," I said. "I want to just hang out with my friends."

Recently, my mom found my passport from those years. I still look at my photograph sometimes, trying to see something, trying to understand who that person was, and maybe who she has become. We are all an accretion of experiences, like silt at the bottom of a lake, our selves constantly writing new selves on top of the old. What could I see in an old passport photo, and in years and years of diaries?

In the photo, one side of my head is shaved, and despite the wide smile, this was at around the time I was done with work; for a short while, at least, I wanted the kind of life any thirteen-year-old had. I wanted to make bad decisions; I wanted to smoke cigarettes. I just wanted to listen to the Cure. (Duran Duran were *so* last year.)

So I quit.

My mom said, "Okay, I'll call your agent."

Proud of my newfound status as "just a kid," I went upstairs to my room. But quickly, the panic set in. Working was my stability, and it was quickly becoming my whole world. Just twenty minutes later, I ran back downstairs.

"Don't call my agent," I said. "I'm good."

I'm sure my mom had been downstairs just waiting me out—she knew me. And that was that. I worked from then on, until the day after *Dead to Me* wrapped.

At age eleven, I'd gotten a dancing job in a Nestea commercial, directed by a big-time British movie director. A young David Arquette was an extra in the same ad. I was dressed in a sweatshirt in the cut-off,

Flashdance, Jennifer Beals kind of way. (Jennifer had invented this look when she had wanted to take off her sweatshirt but didn't want to mess up her hair, instead messing up a generation's worth of perfectly good sweatshirts.)

During the filming of the ad, I was asked to suck on a straw thrust into the iced tea. As we were dancing, the director said to me, "Suck the straw more sexily."

I froze. The director was trying to get me to be more into what I was doing, to more obviously enjoy sipping on the drink, but to a child who had been molested, I heard something else. I had come from somewhere else; I felt uncomfortable around men. I'm not even sure he meant anything by it, but what was an eleven-year-old supposed to do about it?

My work ethic taught me to push through, always. You can't be a blubbering mess when you go to work. Ever since I was a kid, I knew you couldn't bring your shit to set. And because I went to work so early—usually because we didn't have a babysitter, so Mom would take me to whatever set she was on—that professionalism was ingrained from the very start; it's just how it was.

And never once have I ever wished I *hadn't* been a performer. Because if I hadn't?

I'd have been dead. I've watched my friends struggle their whole lives because of how we were raised in that Canyon, but I always had work, always had some place to go. I had an appointment to be somewhere, to prepare for something and to show up and do something. Other people were relying on me, and because I'm an abider of rules, I turned up. I worked, and I sucked it up, and I went back the next day.

Otherwise, coming from where I came from? Not just addicted. Dead for sure.

Work was discipline.

The day after my thirteenth birthday, alongside other thirteen-year-old accounts of my special day and my friends and a Christmas parade we'd all attended, I'd written in my diary, *"PS. I still love Scott."*

I was about to head to my grandmother's house in South Bend for a week. That Christmas we had made our usual trek to South Bend to see her. For some reason, my then boyfriend, Scott, flew in, too.

My previously adoring tone quickly changed, though. At some point during the visit, according to my diary, *"That's when I had to give my first blow job."* It's a tragic indictment that I felt I "had" to do that, and yes, no great surprise, it was terrible. It happened on my grandmother's couch, and frankly, that act was the grossest thing I've ever experienced in my life. As soon as it was over, I felt myself starting to throw up, so I ran to the kitchen and I drank an entire diet soda, just to get the taste out of my mouth. Sex was no surprise to me, but still, it grossed me out. I'd been molested and abused as a young child, and I'd already seen plenty of porn. By the time I was ten, I had already watched *Deep Throat,* and my friends and I had also watched *Letter to Susan,* a lesbian porn movie just left lying around on VHS at a friend's house. Watching it, I'd feel tingly, and weird, a mixture of unease and unhappiness and something unknown.

It all got to me, seeped under my skin, and it came out in my diary as anger toward Scott: *"Know what? Scott went with me to Grandma's. I hate him. He is the biggest asshole in the whole world. I'm gonna break up with him tonight."*

I never said no, but I can tell from those pages that I wasn't ready, that I'd been pushed into a world I was too young for. Still, I soldiered on, my adult work ethic and responsibilities in tow.

At home in the Canyon, I was part of a misfit group of fatherless kids. We had been smoking since we were nine or ten years old, rolling up our school papers and putting oregano in them. We had seen our parents do it, whether with joints or cigarettes. It was just what we knew. We were scrappy, rough around the edges, a bit wild, but never really bad.

My shaved head made casting directors think I was tough, though, and after small roles in various movies and TV shows, I landed a plum character on a show called *Heart of the City*—a cop drama about an L.A. detective raising two kids on his own. I played Robin Kennedy, and even though the show was canceled after one season—we were up against *The Golden Girls* on a Saturday night, which was death to ratings—I still managed to win a Young Artist Award for Exceptional Performance by a Young Actress in a New Television Comedy or Drama Series.

While I was working on *Heart of the City,* something happened that grew to have an outsize effect on my life. What others might have taken as just another innocuous comment became for me a Mount Rushmore–size moment of shame. What that friend said, and what I felt it exposed, ended up setting a precedent for my life that has caused me untold pain.

I don't hold that friend responsible—after all, who knows which words we say or things we do might dramatically affect those around us? She could not have known that three words would set me on a course that would lead directly to me being unable to bask in the successes I've been lucky enough to have had in my career. So much so that it is hard for me to even talk about my work in this book; the thought that anything I say might be construed as bragging fills me with a quiet terror. Deep down I'm proud of what I've done, of pushing past the deprivations of my life and having a successful career, but I'll be damned if I'll say that out loud.

And here's why: I had made it clear to one of my dearest friends that I never wanted to brag about what was happening to me professionally. The phrase I used was, "Tell me if I ever get weird with what I'm doing." And I meant it—I didn't want to be one of those people who thought that my job as an actor somehow signified that I was special. We actors can get so self-regarding, as though the act of inhabiting a character that is different from ourselves is some kind of alchemy, when in fact it's a trade, as mystical and mysterious as knowing how to cut hair or unclog a sink.

Acting for me had always been a job of survival; acting was how my family ate. Just because there were cameras and audiences didn't mean that what I did was necessarily hallowed or rarefied. I knew the techniques required to be funny, for example—that didn't mean I had the keys to cosmic comedy. I just understood where the beats of a line needed to go, the correct timing, the most effective way to hit the right inflection. But it wasn't like I was splitting the atom or saving lives in an emergency room.

So even by my early teens, I meant it when I said,

"Tell me if I ever get weird with what I'm doing." But I was about to be caught up short by that plea. One day my friend and I were on Pico when I realized with a start that we were passing by the 20th Century Fox lot where I was filming *Heart of the City*. We'd been chatting and I hadn't been paying attention, and I remember vividly that the Doors were playing on the car stereo, so my mind was on the music. But echoing the entry on the title page of my journal—business address: "20th Cen Fox"—I innocently said, "Oh my god, that's so weird. That's where I live!"

There was a beat of silence.

"You're doing it," my friend said.

My blood stopped. And that was it. *Tell me if I ever get weird with what I'm doing.* I had gotten weird; I had broken a sacred inner rule to never come off as someone who thought that acting was anything special.

Since that day, I have never spoken again about my accomplishments. Not a single day. I don't boast because that girl whispered in my ear, and still whispers every day, "You're doing it."

But it's not a searing modesty. It's much worse than that. I'm not just desperate to play down my career: in fact I've often felt great shame for doing what I do. Being busted for doing the exact thing I always promised I wouldn't left a taste in my mouth I can't get rid of. The shame is like a virus, hooking onto my low self-esteem and leaving me struggling to gain pleasure in my work. You see my sad eyes? Now maybe you're starting to get why.

When a new show, originally called *Not the Cosbys* (oh, the irony) but retitled *Married... with Children,* was casting, they too wanted a tough, rough-around-the-edges, blue-collar kid to play the character Kelly Bundy, the daughter of a blue-collar slob and a live-wire, blowsy woman. (As originally conceived, Kelly was not a dumbass: she was a biker chick.)

Too many young women coming up in Hollywood since childhood experience unwanted attention and abuse within the industry, but I was lucky to avoid it. I'll never really know why, of course, and we need to stop talking about what women can do and talk more about how men can stop. But I've always had a hunch that being scary was one of the ways I was able to avoid the kind of sexual assaults perpetrated by all those guys who have been exposed in the last few years. My attitude was always — and here I'm quoting myself — "I'm not going to tickle your winky for a job." That was *not* my jam, thank you very much.

It went further than making sure they knew I wasn't going to be railroaded into doing something I didn't want to do: I wasn't going to be nice to people just for the sake of it either. I always felt that I should get a job from merit, not because of my personality. So those fuckers who thought intimidation, be it sexual or otherwise, was the currency knew not to screw with me from the get-go. I didn't play that game; I made them scared of me. Harvey Weinstein, for example, was definitely afraid of me. Once, at a Miramax party, I heard him being lascivious about a woman as she passed by, and before I could even think, I said, "Oh, come on, man. That's just gross." Weinstein just kind of looked at me, and I could tell he was thinking, *Don't talk to me like that.* But at the same time, I could sense a different kind of appraisal, as though he was also thinking, *This chick doesn't fuck around.* And he was right to be afraid of me. I did not fuck around.

From an early age my mom had told me that people in the business needed me more than I needed them. And that stuck with me. It got me through whenever I was being pressured.

When it came to *Married... with Children,* I didn't care either way, though. I read the script and thought it was trash. To me, and to my mom, it read like a bunch of poorly written potty humor. Not the Cosbys, and certainly not for me, thankyouverymuch.

Gosh, I'm getting fat! I have gained so much weight...

As my career on TV blossomed, so did my struggles with body image. By February 15, 1985, when I wrote those words about myself, I was working on a comedy called *Washingtoon*. The pressures of being onscreen had played into my already low self-esteem, creating a tremendously painful and damaging sense that I needed to be as skinny as possible. There are more references to my weight than pretty much anything else in my diaries at around this time. I didn't write much about the roles I was doing. Even at thirteen, working on TV was a job rather than anything notable.

So I'll state for the record that in *Washingtoon* I played a character with the entirely believable name Sally Forehead (at least it wasn't Fivehead, I suppose). Sally was the bratty daughter of an idealistic DC politician in an era — the Reagan years — so long ago and comparatively innocent that politicians could be both harmless figures of fun while at the same time committed to trying to make people's lives better. I know, can you imagine? Now audiences would laugh at the show's ridiculousness instead of at, well, its jokes. You need to watch only a few minutes of *Washingtoon* to see how far our political culture has fallen. The characters might have been buffoons, but they were endearingly earnest. The world that show depicted feels as close to modern politics as to the Roman Senate.

And there I am, with my Thompson Twins haircut,

shaved on the side and all kinds of crazy on top, wearing long, dangly, mid-eighties earrings, gently ribbing my father about the charade that is his job.

I'm as wiry and slim as any thirteen-year-old might be, and yet my diary continually harps on my appearance. Even though *Washingtoon* was short-lived, I was now firmly in the public eye, and that pressure was taking a huge toll. By June 2, 1985, I was writing this in my diary.

> *I'm turning into a vegetarian... I've got to lose weight. I'm becoming a fat blob. I look at myself in the mirror and I see a vision of obesity and blubber. Anyway, I hope I become anorexic.*

I'd been struggling with these kinds of thoughts for years, and though no one moment can lead to a lifetime's affliction, one incident in particular still weighs heavy on my heart. When I was eight years old, one of the neighborhood kids poked at my leg and said, "You're fat." I can trace my obsession with my appearance to that comment, though so many other factors led me to be predisposed to that terrible Irish illness, Ann O'Rexia. I was the child who had been surrounded by abuse. I lived in the public eye. I grew up in a city obsessed with appearance. I craved control in a childhood that had none. All these things made that kid's comment land hard—they were the kindling just waiting for the spark of cruelty.

So began a lifelong struggle with body image and weight, a horrible relationship with food, and a warped sense of self, so bad that I'd spend the rest of my life with a rampant dysmorphia. I never saw the skinny girl everyone else did. I only ever saw something else, and I still do.

As 1985 went on, my issues with weight grew only more pressing, more dire.

> *I'm really down on myself and my body... I have decided to not eat anything and to just drink water and such (other liquids). I feel that in no time at all I will be the skinniest of all my friends, and people will like me more. I strive to be beautiful, but nothing seems to work. My mom said that I might be able to suck the fat out of my thighs. It's a new form of plastic surgery and it is great. I just hope that I can do it soon. The only problem is I might have to be full-grown and maybe I am or maybe I'm not, but I still hope I can do it no matter what it costs. Let's have a toast to being skinny and me getting the fat sucked out.*

It breaks my heart to read this now. The extremity of it all scares me—the pressure I must have felt as an actor to conform to the weird Hollywood "perfection," not to mention that I was already conflating being thin with being liked. No one pointed out that I was dangerously skinny, that my idea of self was warped and I did not need to change myself further. In fact, it was the opposite.

I was a young woman on the precipice of adulthood whose body was already her greatest enemy, not her ally. My mother, all too knowledgeable about the pressures of being a woman, had seemingly done enough research to give me damaging ideas about how to brutalize myself with liposuction, how to reach for a "perfection" that was neither obtainable nor even real. I was thirteen. I can only imagine that this was a projection of her own struggles, of a bond that went beyond mother and child into something closer, intermingled in ways that were both more meaningful and more codependent.

It would take me years to understand that "perfect" was a chimera, a falsehood, and a life-threatening falsehood at that. That I could be a size 0 and call myself a "fat blob" signaled the failure of so many things: my own ability to see clearly, my mother's guidance, the culture of not just Hollywood but the wider world. Was it any wonder that when I looked in the mirror, I saw not beauty but the opposite?

* * *

Still, I saw beauty in others. I had been fortunate to meet a girl on the set of *Charles in Charge* named Samantha Smith, who stood out as an incredible role model.

I had appeared in two episodes of the first season of *Charles in Charge*, which was then a smash hit show. In one I'd taped—episode 6, "Slumber Party"—Samantha had also appeared, playing one of the girls who shows up for the party. (Each of the girls arrives with something to contribute to the evening's fun. One brought a poster of Simon Le Bon from Duran Duran and I can only imagine that was my idea.)

Samantha was already famous before her brief cameo on *Charles in Charge*. In November 1982, she had written a simple letter to the then leader of the Soviet Union, Yuri Andropov. In the letter, she had revealed to the Russian premier her fears about a nuclear war between the U.S. and the Soviets, imploring him to commit to avoiding a catastrophe. Andropov eventually wrote back; on the back of his very public response, Samantha had become a symbol of hope for the two Cold War superpowers, had subsequently spent two weeks in Russia, and had become a significant celebrity on her return stateside.

When she and I met, none of that really mattered. We were just two sharp kids working on a TV show, and we quickly became firm friends; she was sweet and interesting and wise beyond her years.

Then one day I was sitting on the steps outside the

set of *Washingtoon*, having a cigarette, when someone found me to deliver the news.

"Can you believe that little girl who wrote that letter to the Soviets just died in a plane crash?"

My heart stopped, and my head fell into my hands. There had been a crash in Maine as Samantha had been returning home from shooting a TV show, and she and her father, along with four other passengers and two crew, had died.

I couldn't breathe. One of the older actors on *Washingtoon*, seeing me crying, asked me what had happened. I could barely get the words out.

"My friend just died," I said.

The actor took out a piece of yellow paper, and with a blue pen he wrote, "Here's to the tears of friendship. May they crystallize as they fall and be worn as gems in the memory of those we love."

I still have that piece of paper.

I sometimes turn to my journals from back then to try to connect with Samantha. I can hear my fourteen-year-old self in the exclamation points and emotion on the page.

May 17, 1986
Fuck she was special. I miss her!!!!!... I am

scared that if I get too depressed, I might kill myself. Which is something I don't really want to do, but when I throw a frenzy, I am capable of any kind of destruction to myself.

June 12, 1986
I hate this world!!!! The other day at school, I tried to kill myself. I just wish I would have succeeded! Every day seems to get worse. Dying sounds better and better. Ever since Samantha's death things haven't been too good... Fuck I miss her! I just want to be with her. My sweetheart. My love. Her picture is on my wall looking over me like a guardian angel.

I want to go back and find that fourteen-year-old girl, the one who was determined to be modest to the point of self-effacement, the one struggling with her body image, the one fasting, drinking only water, the girl who had survived so much and who now had to deal with the violent loss of her friend. I want to wrap her up so tightly and tell her everything will be okay.

I often think about how MS is exacerbated by trauma. My current stomach problems act up if someone starts to stress me out. I start vomiting, almost like my body is trying to stop the noise, too. Then I end up in the hospital again.

I just want everything to stop.

But it won't stop. I'll be stuck in this bed, my brain lesions sparking like a downed wire. I'll be poring through my journals from when I was young, trying to find the key to something. Perhaps I saw into the future in ways that are hard to believe. This from, again, June 1986.

> *The bright days that I so looked forward to are turning to gray. Why is life for me more of a chore than an experience? Each time I awake I dread the day that will follow. I wish that the pain I feel inside would terminate. I hate it here. But I suppose that I should "look on the bright side." My heart says what bright side and my mind says that there is joy on the "long and winding road" ahead. I just don't know if I should follow that road. Who knows what it's leading to. Either happiness or sadness. I think that I should just give it a try.*

I suppose I did follow that road, but did it lead to happiness or sadness?

Just as for everyone, for me it led to both. It led me here.

You with the Sad Eyes

* * *

With everything turning to gray, I thought comedy was beneath me. My world was punk and the Canyon and Melrose and three hours of school every few weeks between jobs. Committing to a comedy show like *Married... with Children,* which was billed as an antidote to the smarmy charms of *The Cosby Show*?

No thanks—comedy was for suckers. I had a shaved head and a gnarly attitude.

I was sure that I was destined for a career filled with dramatic roles, like the one I'd won an award for on *Heart of the City.* Comedy was so not what I was.

I hated myself.

And I hated Kelly Bundy.

But there was more—the hair band generation as depicted in the character of Kelly? It was so not my thing, so not my style. *I was from the Canyon, from Joni-land. Stephen Stills was my godfather.* By fifteen, I'd discovered Janis Joplin and I rued the fact that I'd missed Woodstock every day. I wore patchouli, which some people told me meant I smelled like goat BO. (They were not wrong.) I was the child of a *real* hippie. I was not comedy; I was not Kelly Bundy.

Some days my friends and I would walk all the way down to Melrose from Lookout Mountain. Back then,

Melrose was a scene. There were clothing stores like Aaardvark's, grimy and grungy and awesome. Those stores smelled like crack. Sure enough, I found out later that a friend of a friend was smoking crack in the back of one of them. Out on the street, homeless teenagers slept and waited and begged for change. They were mostly runaways, or kids who had been kicked out of their homes. There they were, lounging around on Melrose with their mohawks, in tattered clothes covered in zippers, smoking cigarettes and waiting for something good to happen. It felt like we were all punks back then: on Melrose, at Aaardvark's, in the alleys sniffing glue, at Fairfax High School, where the Red Hot Chili Peppers would come from one day soon.

I didn't go to Fairfax HS. I went to Excelsior HS, just off of Highland Avenue in the very heart of Hollywood.

Excelsior was a school for working kids. We went there from 9 a.m. till noon only, leaving us plenty of time to do our real jobs.

Excelsior claimed to be a "college prep" school. In reality, it was so lax that we would regularly get away with changing the clocks so the head of the school would think we were done for the day. He'd go to the bathroom or to the office, and we'd immediately nominate someone to go up and move the hands of the clock to read noon. When he returned, he'd look at the clock and announce, "Ah, looks like we're done!" He was probably as relieved as we were.

It was a weird little school. There were only about thirty of us in the student body at any one time. I went to school with people like Corey Haim, Corey Feldman, and Milla Jovovich, as well as a bunch of kids who had to work for their parents in the afternoons in stores, restaurants, and other family businesses. Originally, I had tried going to Taft High School out in Woodland Hills because my manager lived there and all the high schools down in Hollywood sucked—Hollywood High and Fairfax were scary places to go in the early eighties. I lasted at Taft for one week, and every day I was there I thought I was going to lose my mind. I'd never seen so many cheerleaders and what the character John Bender in *The Breakfast Club* describes as "Sportos" in my life. I was horrified by these people. I would wear pillowcases as skirts with fishnets and Doc Martens. I was a messy, weird, punk chick who, when I started on *Married...with Children*, was making $20,000 a week. Normal high school culture was not for me.

I made the switch to Excelsior, which was more my people, and anyway, it was also the kind of place where you didn't have to go every day if you had a job—they would send you home with the schoolwork, which you'd then just hand in to a tutor, if you did it at all.

A typical month for me would consist of three weeks on an acting job, and then during the week that we had hiatus I'd go back to Excelsior. That was my routine right through eleventh grade.

All I wanted was to get my GED.

Alas, all I ended up with was a high school equivalency.

To complete my high school education, I drove myself to a test center in my white Honda Accord. It was a piece of shit car, but I'd named her Pearl after Janis Joplin. The day of the test was one of those fall days, the leaves starting to come down, the air crisp and bright. I was so excited. I still get butterflies when I think about that moment, the drive there and the way the sun was hitting the leaves and reflecting on the ground, the rest of my life just waiting on the edge of this feeling. Though I probably couldn't have expressed it then, I knew something big, life-changing, was on the horizon—I could feel it in the way the weather was filled with possibility and spark.

I went into the test center and found myself surrounded by a bunch of pregnant girls. We were taking a test that some of us would never need—I sure as shit knew I didn't need it, even though I was a straight A student—and a lot of those young women were about to have something way more important to deal with. As for me, I was already a full-time actor. All I had to really do was sign my name, sit there for a couple of hours, get my certificate, and then... what, exactly?

Oh, I also remember that they asked me if I had any income.

By the end of high school, I sure did.

Oh, and I wasn't pregnant. In fact, I was a virgin.

I'd come to find out that comedy is one of the hardest types, if not *the* hardest type, of acting. For it to be effective, you have to perform as though you're working on the biggest drama in the world, but then you've got to twinkle above it, turning up the volume into another realm. It's crucial to find the right level for that twinkle dial: if you turn the dial too high, then you veer off into camp. Certain movies call for camp, like *Anchorman*, but for subtle humor, the dial's got to be at a two, not a ten. You have to work comedy the same way you would anything else. It takes taste, and skill, and care, and a kind of reserve so you don't descend into something garish.

I'd turned down *Married...*, so the pilot featured another kid in the role of Kelly, but it just didn't work, so they came back to me. The casting director sent me a VHS of the pilot, and my mom and I reluctantly watched it one evening. I'm not sure what we thought we'd see, or why we even watched it in the first place, as I was dead set against it. Boy, how much we wanted to hate it... We sat there like two little snotty actory assholes who'd spent their lives doing Shakespeare.

And then, as the show played, we realized we could not stop laughing.

I looked at my mom. She looked at me.

"Fuck!" I said. "It's funny. It's good. It's really dirty and good." Mom just nodded; I think she knew we'd been given a gift.

I came down from my high horse and accepted the part. The producers had me come to a studio in Burbank to do a "chemistry read." I hate that phrase; it makes me want to throw up when someone uses it, including me. Whoever is the best person for the job is the right person for the role—you can hate someone and still do a great job. Debra Winger and Richard Gere famously didn't like each other when they made *An Officer and a Gentleman,* but they fucked like two rabbits in heat (in the movie, that is). But there, acting opposite me, was David Faustino. David and I hit it off so well in that read, and that was that. They had hoped that David and I were the team. It was almost like they knew it all along.

Now I knew it, too.

FIVE

MARRIED... WITH CHILDREN

Love,
Christina Applegate
(just practicing!)

By the middle of September 1986, I was practicing signing my name for fans. Thank god my friend who'd busted me for my attitude as we passed Fox that day wasn't privy to my diaries.

I had been regularly working for my entire childhood, but as I approached fifteen, perhaps some part of me recognized that a new kind of fame—the kind of fame where autographs would be asked for and granted—was just around the corner. Sure, I'd done a whole bunch of TV shows, but I could still walk the streets of Los Angeles without anyone recognizing me.

All that was about to change.

The first episode of *Married...with Children* aired on April 5, 1987. The show wasn't a hit out of the gate—Fox was then a brand-new channel, joining ABC, CBS, and NBC (imagine: just four stations!), and it was years away from being the juggernaut it is these days. I don't think any of us thought the show itself would still be going a decade later, and the early, snobbish reviews hardly helped. Most of them focused on what was perceived to be the show's crudity, broadness of humor, misogyny, and obsession with sex.

Loved by critics or not, I was suddenly on a major TV show and quickly became paid accordingly. I started at twenty grand per show, which for a fifteen-year-old was a lot of money (it was a lot for anyone, and it still is). I already owned that house behind the Country Store in Laurel Canyon, the one the early radio ads had funded, but now my bank account swelled with network cash.

But money wouldn't solve everything. By January 1988, the negative aura around the show, and my lingering superiority complex when it came to comedy, was evident in my diary entries. That month I wrote, "I'll show these fuckers that I ain't no comedy bullshit actress...," and "I need to do a *movie*. I like it so much more than this fucking comedy live-audience bullshit. Comedy is all timing and line readings. I hate that."

Despite my teenage angst, the set itself was a formative place to work because it was all professional all the time—few allowances were made for my tender age, and I respected that. I remember being sick with a 103-degree fever one day. I was lying on the famous couch and said to a nearby stage manager, "Can you please get me some orange juice?"

She said simply but not unkindly, "You have legs."

Message received. I never asked anybody for anything ever again, to the point where years later, when I was working eighteen hours a day because I was the central character, and in every scene, of the sitcom *Samantha Who?*, I was still running off to get my own coffee, until a PA finally stopped me.

"Can you please stop going to craft services?" he said. "You're actually taking time away from set." Still, it hurt every bit of myself to ask him to get me my double espresso. (I was so tired I was drinking ten or more every day just to get through.)

So *Married...* was where I truly grew up. It was a place of do it for yourself, a place to be professional, to be on time, to know your lines, and everyone else's, to hit your marks. There was no fucking about—ever. (Let it also be noted that my mother came to every single taping across all eleven years.) It may have looked like a loosey-goosey comedy, but as I've said, comedy doesn't work unless it's tight, choreographed, nailed.

We nailed it every single week.

* * *

Though Kelly Bundy was supposed to be a tough biker chick, that changed quickly. A short time after the show began, I happened to go to the Cinerama Dome on Sunset Boulevard to watch a documentary called *The Decline of Western Civilization Part II: The Metal Years*. In the movie, documentarian Penelope Spheeris heads to Gazzarri's, a nightclub on the Sunset Strip, to chat with a young woman named Cindy Birmisa, aka Miss Gazzarri Dancer 1987. Cindy had just won that prestigious competition, a contest in which girls wearing Lycra dresses, their hair way up, super big, all crimped and groupie-like, dance and twerk for their suppers, all hoping to win that cherished title.

At one point, Spheeris asks Miss Gazzarri, "What are you going to do now?," and without missing a beat, Ms. Birmisa answers, "I'm going to continue on with my modeling and hopefully go on with my actressing."

The next morning, I called production and the wardrobe people on *Married*...

"Kelly Bundy is someone else now. We're going down to Melrose. We're going to get some concho belts. We're going to get Lycra dresses. We're going to go full rock slut."

Kelly Bundy was going to do some actressing.

The transformation was immediate, and iconic. Kelly Bundy now exuded a kind of innocent sexiness. She was fully recognizable as an eighties icon, a lovable airhead who hung out with wannabe rock stars.

You with the Sad Eyes

If you watch *Married... with Children* closely, you'll see pretty quickly that I played Kelly as a tease, and as a virgin—which is why I think viewers loved her rather than hated her. One of the creators, Michael Moye, and I talked about this regularly. We agreed to keep Kelly virginal and have the "Kelly is a tramp" opinion come solely from her brother, Bud. In season 2, Bud says, "You're dirt, Kel." When I watch this now, it rings so harshly and makes Bud seem despicable to me. But in the episode, I reply, "Yes, but everybody knows it!," taking the wind out of his misogynist sails. Kelly knew what people thought of her and wasn't fazed by it because we all knew, or should have known, it wasn't true. (And yet, alas, in that same episode I'm wearing a tight leather skirt and wiggling my ass to put the other bowlers off in a bowling tournament.)

That said, Kelly was never overtly promiscuous. Bud might have accused her of it, but she gave no indication that she did much beyond flirting. She was a product of the time, of MTV music videos, with women who wore corsets that were way too tight and did weird stuff for guys with frizzy hair. At the time, these videos were everywhere, and it was my way of expressing what was happening in the zeitgeist. Yet I have been told that I just played a whore. Not true.

Kelly was important to me, and I needed to be perfect for her. I'd shaped the role, and I would damn well put my all into it. I dug myself into a hole with that character, though, because I had to be skinny. I had a vision of the specific clothes I wanted her to wear, and to wear those clothes, I had to lean even deeper into my eating disorder.

The anorexia was terrible. I wanted my bones to be sticking out. If I did eat something, I'd punish myself. Sometimes I wouldn't eat for a whole day.

My diary from those days recounts the deepening of my self-image torture, through both prose and poetry. On TV I was playing a kind of dumb-blonde, Miss Gazzarri Dancer role, but in private I was writing poetry and dressing grungily, slathered in patchouli oil like a little hippie weirdo. In fact, my diary from 1987 reveals a sixteen-year-old who, though now increasingly famous, was still deeply conflicted, struggling, and often in emotional agony.

There's a poem from that time titled "Help Me I'm Falling," a reference to the Joni Mitchell song "Help Me."

> *The sea is not a sea*
> *A tree is not a tree.*
> *It has all gone away.*
> *I cannot see.*
> *The walls are closing in*
> *I don't know where I've been*
> *My life has lost its light*
> *There comes nothing from within.*
> *I only am alone*

You with the Sad Eyes

I only am one
There is no one else
God, what have I done
There was once a shining star
I don't know where you are
You have all burnt out
You have traveled oh so far
Not that there is nothing
The bride has thrown the ring
The moon is black
I'm a bird without a wing

The surrounding pages are filled with the pain of a young woman whose traumatic childhood was catching up with her.

I feel there is something missing. I don't know what, but something. I feel cluttered, I feel lonely. I feel claustrophobic…
 I'm losing weight but I can't see it. I'm getting compulsive about it though. I mean I'm not puking my food up or anything. But I'm afraid to eat and I shouldn't eat. I just don't want to gain it back… I want to change my appearance completely. I hate to look at myself anymore. I'm bored with everything about me. My hair, face, body. I want auburn hair right above my breasts. I

want a defined face. I want to be beautiful. But now I'm too plain. I'm not ugly, but I'm not anything exciting. I will blow them away with my portrayal of a nympho on Jump Street though. So ha, ha, motherfuckers.

In 1987, I had indeed booked a guest spot on *21 Jump Street,* another hit Fox show. It was being filmed in Vancouver rather than L.A., and it would be the series that made Johnny Depp's name. I already knew Johnny: he was part of my friend group growing up, a group that included my still-best friend, Sam Sarkar. Sam has been there for me in every conceivable way since I was fifteen years old. He's seen me at my best, and my worst; my mom always said I should have married him. But it's for the best that I didn't, because he's one of my closest friends and I know he always will be.

One thing is very clear from the journals: I was in love with Johnny Depp for years. He was eight years older than me. He always behaved impeccably toward me, even though I was clearly mad about him. It seems that back then I was just one of the guys to him, yet my journals are filled with complicated and ever-changing feelings. I swing from swoon to a cold bucket of water on the face in the span of less than two months.

> *I've been having really strange dreams about Johnny of all people. I can't really analyze them because I don't remember what they are once I wake up. I can only remember who's in them...Johnny...*
>
> *...*
>
> *I can't sit here and wish he was something that he's not. I can't change him. But yet I wish I could get through to him.*

Johnny and his guy friends would invite me up to Vancouver to hang out with them while he was filming *21 Jump Street*. There are lots of entries about my trips to Canada in my journals; mostly, I loved it up there with the guys. I would sleep in the same bed as my friend Sam—he would never try to touch me, nor me him, which is why we're still best friends to this day. In the morning, he would make coffee and put a little Baileys Irish Cream in it and we would talk and write poetry.

One incident from those days is notably missing from my journals.

On one trip to Vancouver, I went to hang out with Kim Manners, a longtime TV guy who directed a bunch of episodes of *Jump Street*, at his place out in the woods surrounding the city. I remember sitting, dangling my legs into the hot tub, and then my memory turns to total darkness. Everything is missing until I found myself scrambling up some stairs, with no idea where I was. I frantically searched for a piece of mail or anything with an address on it. Finally, I called a cab. It dropped me off back where I had been staying with the guys. I didn't tell anyone what had happened; I kept my cards close to my chest.

I had marks all over my butt, but that's all I knew. Clearly, something bad had happened, but to this day I have no idea the full extent of it, though it's not hard to imagine what that guy did to me.

I remember Sam putting me to bed and looking after me. Sam was, and still is, my angel.

Orbiting in and out of this group was a little-known actor named Brad Pitt. In 1989, I invited him to be my date at the MTV Video Music Awards. He was already a part of my extended friend group—we had been platonic pals for the longest time. He'd often swing by my 750-square-foot row house with the tiny door, and we'd have barbecues and hang out, always as part of a bigger group. Sometimes he and Sam would do a little gardening—I still have pictures of them with rakes in their hands, cleaning up my mom's yard.

Then one day I took another look at Brad and thought, *Hmm*... Apparently, he did the same, and so

I invited him to the awards. I had to get there early to rehearse my appearance, and Brad was kind enough to drive to my house to pick up my mom and Lori Depp and get them to the theater. In my 1988 journal I note, "My best friend is Johnny's ex-wife Lori, pretty scary, huh?" (Johnny and Lori had been married for three years in the mid-eighties.)

That night I was to present the Best Group Video award alongside Alice Cooper. I was peak Kelly Bundy at that point, at least as far as the outside world saw it—even the script I'd been handed played into my dumb blonde persona. As we introduced the nominees, I was to ask Alice, "No solo artist has ever won in this category—coincidence or conspiracy? What do you think?," to which he was to reply, "Christina, you're *such* a Bundy."

But I was something else, too, at least in my own mind. Far from an idiot in a Lycra dress or cropped T-shirt, I'd chosen a Ceil Chapman gown to wear for that MTV show. Friends told me it wasn't appropriate for that kind of evening. It was too classy, too classic, too 1950s, too Old Hollywood. Chapman was a legendary designer of the forties and fifties—she dressed Marilyn Monroe, Greer Garson, Elizabeth Taylor, and many others—and to get the dress, we had to punch in a secret code at the atelier, and then agree not to touch any of the garments housed there unless we intended to buy them, so rare and expensive were they.

That Chapman dress is a one-of-a-kind — I still have it. I forget exactly how much I paid for it, but I know it was a lot. Diaphanous and ethereal, it boasts large red and yellow and black hand-drawn flowers on a white shift, and I paired it with a scarf of the same material wrapped around my blond hair. I think it's the single best dress I've ever worn in my life. I felt incredible in it, and no, it wasn't the kind of thing the MTV awards expected, and no, I didn't give a shit. That dress was me, expressed perfectly.

In fact, I felt so powerful and sure of myself for once that when the awards show was over, I left with Sebastian Bach, *not* Brad Pitt. I had spent all night staring at Bach, who was then a long-haired hunk fronting the band Skid Row. I hate to put it like this, but Brad back then was still making his way as an actor, and he wasn't yet THE Brad Pitt, the man of so many people's dreams.

And it gets worse: Brad was left to sullenly drive my mom and Lori home. Apparently, at a gas station on the way, Brad almost got into a fight with a bunch of gang members, and, not surprisingly, was subsequently very mad at me. We didn't talk for many years after that. Much later, but at different times, two of his movie star girlfriends asked me if it was true that I was the girl who left Brad behind at the MTV Video Music Awards. Brad had apparently told both of them separately that he was still mad at me. Eventually, we agreed that I'd been a kid, and though he'd deserved much better, it was time to forgive the child who dumped him for the lead singer of Skid Row.

Of course, Brad is now THE Brad Pitt, and Sebastian Bach...well, he still has long hair, I guess. My diary at the time doesn't exactly reek with guilt—I was a seventeen-year-old television star in a Chapman dress. It seems Bach and I ended up at Cathouse, the notorious once-a-week club where people danced to rock music, where Guns N' Roses, Mötley Crüe, Aerosmith, and so many others would hang out.

> *Friday, September 8, 1989*
> *Wow, what a couple of days I've had. I did the MTV awards on Wednesday and had such a blast. I met every famous groovy person imaginable. Then I went to a couple of parties, ended up at Cathouse with Sebastian Bach.*

Alas, no mention of Brad *at all*. Oops. It wasn't as if Bach was a catch in any case, and yet I still found myself worrying about *his* feelings more than my own, a fatal flaw that I carry with me to this day.

> *I'm feeling extremely lonely right now. I feel out of control. Sebastian has a 1-year-old child. What a dick. Why do I always attract the "winners." I had really started to like*

him. I mean, I wouldn't want a relationship with him or anything, but still the whole thing is that he did that having a kid. Spent the night at my house and befriended me. Thank god I didn't have sex with him; that would have been horrible. I feel extremely out of touch right now. It's freaking me. I had two days of living in the fast lane and shit it's fun but shouldn't be done a lot. You really lose touch with your morals… I hate the whole famous thing and the whole "scene" for that matter. Wow, I can't wait to see what the magazines have to say about all of this. The rumors are probably flying about Sebastian and me right now. But I don't know what to do. I really want to go to his show on Sunday but if I tell him [that I know about his child] I can't; he might get really upset and that's not good. Especially before a gig. But then if I do go, I can't tell him I know before he goes on because that would be confrontation. So I'd have to wait till afterwards which means a couple of hours of torture beforehand…

My ability to catch the eye of a then famous rock star and then ditch someone like Brad Pitt at an after-party while wearing a one-of-a-kind Ceil Chapman dress still couldn't convince me I was an attractive person. Even after I found out Bach had a long-term partner and a child, for too long, according to my diaries, I wondered if he and I had a future. For millions of Americans watching *Married... with Children,* I was an exemplar of female beauty, but to me I was "too plain." I thought my face was mediocre at best. I worked on my body so hard, but I was never satisfied. There were days when I'd go to a spin class and then work out with my trainer and then go to a dance class for two and a half more hours, always chasing the unobtainable, abusing my body in the service of a quest for perfection that was itself as damaging as any addiction. My sickness for perfection was always the driving force in my life.

I can't blame anyone on *Married...* for what I went through. Sure, it was always part of the show that I would be an object for men to leer at, but I was the one who wanted to wear those Kelly Bundy dresses to represent something in the zeitgeist. This whole rock-slut thing was happening, and it was completely fascinating to me, and I thought it would be interesting to try to capture it on the show. And as hard as it may be to believe, I was genuinely innocent of my effect on people. I was just a kid.

By season 2, I was still only sixteen years old, and dressing relatively modestly on the show, although there were times I would walk on set and the crowd would catcall me. In episode 3 of that second season, I entered stage left in an off-the-shoulder sea-green dress, and someone audibly whistled from the audience. I was so disconnected from who I was and what I gave off—I had no idea I was attractive to anyone, as multiple entries in my journals will attest—that the catcalling passed me by completely.

And it wasn't just that I didn't expect anyone to actually express lust my way—I was just working, very much focused on the scene and what it needed to be a success, concentrating on landing my lines with the right cadence and timing, hitting my spots, reacting to the other actors in what I hoped was a genuine and convincing way. Just because it's a comedy doesn't mean it should be all about the laughs—you have to get the basics dead-on in comedy, perhaps even more so than in a serious drama. Too much or too little and you miss the mark completely and it stops being funny. I treated this job as I'd treated all the ones that came before. I had to get it right.

And yes, I was truly innocent, and I was very young, so the whooping and hollering? I didn't hear it, even though we always had a live audience, and sometimes they would get so loud and inappropriate that the crew would have to tell them to shut up.

By season 3 all bets were off—by episode 3 of that season I was in a tight purple shirt, my leg up on a table, trying to entice "Matt the football player." More and more my midriff was bare, the clothes tighter, the skirts shorter. By season 5, my god: I can walk into the living room, as I do in episode 13, "The Godfather," in a leather fringed jacket over a short red shirt and there's a five-second break in the scene while the crowd hollers lustily at me.

I look at all this now, and I cringe. The show was indeed broad, and lewd, and it wouldn't have a shot in hell of being made these days. That's a good thing: it's hard enough for young women to thrive in a world of appearances. Just the other day I caught myself pointing out to Sadie how bloated my stomach was, having just gotten home from yet another hospital visit. Immediately, I regretted saying anything at all about appearances to my daughter. I never want anyone, me least of all, to talk about how women look, especially around Sadie. I want people to love her for her smarts, and humor, and charisma, and kindness (all things they do, indeed, love her for). Her physical beauty should be beside the point, so I'm damned if I'm going to echo what the world is already saying too loudly.

Back in the late eighties, the world seemed to think that I, Christina Applegate, not Kelly Bundy, dressed like Miss Gazzarri, too. This suited me greatly because away from the set I could just be me and not be recognized. I could walk through Hollywood and only the keenest of observers would recognize me. Still, every Friday for a taping I had to squeeze into those clothes, clothes that would show if you ate something as tiny as a single grape. If I was going to eat something as horrendously huge as a bagel, say, I would scoop it out and maybe eat only half of it, or maybe half of a half. And that would be my food intake for an entire day.

> *I can't tell if I'm getting fat or not. It truly is becoming an obsession. I am going to be thin. I am destined to be thin. I am THIN!!! I want to be so that people say, "Shit, I wish I could have a body like that." They will if I get my act together.*
>
> *. . .*
>
> *I feel like a cow again. I gained two pounds. I still don't like the direction. I've got to stop eating. I can't help it though. (119 lbs. I want to be 110. Let's see how fast I can do it.)*
>
> *. . .*
>
> *I've gained some weight back that I lost. But see, I don't have a deadline to lose the weight like I did when the dance episode [Season 3, Episode 13] was coming up. I felt so much better then when my stomach was super flat.*

I knew my anger toward myself, my self-denial of food, and my generally damaging relationship with it were all trauma-based. I had seen altogether too much at a young age, and any sense of control and safety was passing at best. Anorexia has been likened to a kind of OCD. When someone makes me feel out of control, I have to reassert that control, and anorexia lets me do that. (She is a bitch, though—she still sometimes sneaks her way in. But I now have the power to tell her to go fuck herself, too.) I've often said that if I could live in a Japanese *minka* with sliding doors, tatami mats, and maybe one bonsai tree, I'd be the happiest person alive. Like many traumatized people, I ache for control, and food is one place I'm able to achieve it.

The week before I turned eighteen, I wrote,

> *Wednesday, November 15, 1989, 11:07 p.m.*
> *What can I say? Once again I feel fat. I think I'm getting a grip on why I do, so often. No guy = fat girl. A guy = skinny, happy girl. Go figure. Then work, hard work = skinny happy girl.*

My diaries list almost endless problems with the men I picked to date. When I was seventeen, for a brief second, I hung out with Anthony Kiedis. I had gone to see the Red Hot Chili Peppers at this weird venue, a Masonic hall or somewhere just like that. I distinctly remember that we all sat on folding chairs, and there was carpet on the floor. At some point my friend told me that the lead singer wanted to say hi to me.

When Anthony found me, he had a top hat on.

"Why are you wearing a top hat?" I said.

"I want to go out with you," he said. That's not why he was wearing the top hat. He had ignored my question.

"Okay," I said, realizing I probably wasn't going to get an answer about the hat.

We planned a date to go to a farmer's market—let me repeat that: Anthony Kiedis and I planned a date at a farmer's market. That's how punk rock we were.

Cut to: I'm sitting at a farmer's market with Anthony and then my mom shows up to pick me up, buys herself a sandwich, and joins us.

My favorite thing that Antoine—that's what we all called him—ever said to me was about how he sometimes avoided using deodorant.

"A horse will know me before they will know you," he said.

I think it's very important to be recognized by horses. Then Antoine dumped me, but right after he did so, he said, "Hey, could you do my laundry?"

And like a stupid fucking fan I did it.

My feeling has always been, "I'm going to fix you. I'm going to save you. I'm going to help you. I have the means to help you. I have the means to save you, and I have the means to fix you." I loved the assholes and fuckups because they were interesting and different and musical and weird.

Many women find men they want to fix, counting on a serial hope that these men will become what we envisage for our lives. Sometimes it's possible, but mostly, ladies, it ain't. My universe always sent me beautifully fucked-up dudes in need of fixing. But maybe I was the one who needed fixing after all.

I was constantly in conflict with men who didn't call me, who played games, who shifted their affections and ignored me. Partly this is because we were all so young, of course, but I also think I was fatally attracted to men who were troubled and selfish and self-centered. (This would come to be very true the older I got.) And somehow, I'd allied my self-worth and my disgust for my own body with the fluctuating attentions of young men who were unserious about relationships, if they thought about them at all.

What I desperately wanted was *control,* and that control was often most fervently needed when I came up against cruel behavior.

A few years after *Married...* ended, I shot a movie in England, and someone in the production crew was so cruel to me, verbally abusing me, that I found myself controlling the situation by yet again severely limiting what went into my body. Most days I would have only soup for lunch. If there was one drop of oil in it, I would push it away, telling myself I couldn't eat it. Some days I would have one bite—one bite!—of a banana, and nothing more. I even had a spin bike installed in my hotel room, and I'd spin all day long. Now, having a daughter and wanting so much for her, it kills me how I treated my young self.

I was down to maybe one hundred pounds, and one day I kept one of my best friends waiting while I did another forty-five minutes on the bike—she had traveled four hours across the UK to see me. When I finished my workout, she said to me, "You look *disgusting.*"

I hadn't even looked in the mirror—I couldn't bear to—so this was news to me. I remember sitting on the toilet that day and looking down at my stomach... only to find I *had* no stomach. All I could see were bones—rib bones, hip bones, bones bones bones. I used to joke back then that if my hip bones weren't the first thing to enter a room, I was overweight.

Married... with Children was the orphaned child of the Fox network—no one really paid attention to us. We were controversial, for sure, especially after the intervention of an anti-obscenity activist, Terry Rakolta, who single-handedly wrote letters to advertisers complaining about "blatant exploitation of women and sex and anti-family attitudes." On the back of her one-woman crusade, we lost a bunch of advertisers—including McDonald's and Procter & Gamble, the latter of which went as far as to say the show was a "negative portrayal of the American family." I didn't know what perfect American family they were talking about. With the controversy swirling, the show got moved from our original 8:30 p.m. slot to 9 p.m., post watershed. But our ratings continued to be solid, and within a year all the advertisers had returned. It's probably worth noting that compared to today's TV, *Married...* was incredibly tame, but we aired in Reagan's America, replete with its rise of the religious right and tut-tutting from the Moral Majority.

I'd love to hear what Ms. Rakolta thinks of sitcoms these days, with their blow job jokes and backdoor fun.

Katey Sagal, who played my mom on the show, had the last laugh, of course. In an interview a couple of years ago she said, "We sent Terry Rakolta flowers every year. She tried to get us off the air and all it did was get us on the front page of the *New York Times*. And it doubled our audience."

Eventually, the show cemented itself into American culture — it was never quite a smash hit, despite Terry Rakolta's best efforts, but it was a cornerstone of Fox's output, and we all became famous in our way. I remember at some point we went to a mall in the middle of somewhere for an appearance, and once we were done, a crowd of fans literally chased us back to our cars. Everyone wanted a piece of us, especially me.

It was our Beatles-at-Shea moment.

I don't remember where the mall was, but Ed O'Neill, who played my dad, and Katey would know—they have the best memories of any two human beings I've ever known in my life. Ed, especially, remembers *everything*.

"Don't you remember?" he'll say. "Come on, Christina!"

"Nope, not a clue," I'll say.

It was a different world. Before Sadie, before my star in Hollywood.

Before MS.

As for Kelly Bundy, well, she just liked the attention; she didn't do anything with it. If she had been one-dimensional, no one would have cared for her. Instead, even when she was being provocative, she was still innocent. At least in the early seasons, she was too young to be sleeping with people.

As for the actor who played Kelly, she waited until the propitious date of 8/8/88 to have sex for the first time, as diligently noted in my diary.

> *Guess what? You know when I was talking about how I needed to have sex? Well, I did. And I did the dirty deed with the only person*

You with the Sad Eyes

I would want to do it for the first time with anyway. I just made love to [name redacted] twice. It hurt like a motherfucker. But oh well, it's over with.

Alas, as with so many people having sex for the first time, it led only to regrets. In the name of romance, I had told the guy, "Just put it in for a second so I know what it feels like." That was my first Sexy Town.

Four days later, I wrote that I had "major regrets about the incident," saying, "I'm glad it's over with but yet I really wish I hadn't done it."

I was stuck between caring about this person and dealing with their lack of care for me, but I brushed it off, internalizing as usual. The "incident" further depleted my self-worth, leading to a swirl of darker poetry. Here's one elegantly named "Drunken Bitch."

*Christina loves someone
But who it is is yet to be decifered
between God and the Devil
But until then I will be left
alone
Here with my dagger and
my heart.
Not knowing what to do with
either.*

Despite the bad decisions and agonies swirling around, the poet in me could still find the beauty in life.

> *Today was yet another beautiful day. It was so clear. Momma, Mariah, and I went to Self-Realization Lake Shrine [in the Palisades]... it was really great. I've totally started to appreciate my life & surroundings this week. Life is really a masterpiece. If you just open your mind and your eyes you can really see how beautiful things are... So when I say "life is shit," I can look back and realize that there is another side. And stop being so skeptical about everything.*

Even at that young age, I didn't want to feel pain. So I dove into work, and into saving people. And spirituality was also a crutch at that time—it helped me get away from the big waves, like the ones on the north shore of Hawaii.

As for Kelly Bundy, well, she was certainly no poet—she seemed to be written as dumber and dumber and dumber. She had started out as a biker chick who liked biker guys, wearing ratted jean jackets and sporting a smart mouth. But as the seasons progressed, her intelligence withered entirely, until the day I was handed a script in which she didn't know how to do something as simple as open a fucking door.

However I felt, being on the show provided all kinds of opportunities for me to expand my career. Earlier in 1989, a few months before I ditched Brad Pitt at the MTV Video Music Awards, I'd attended the February Grammys at the Shrine. I still have the ticket — I was in row 23, seat 49, if you're scoring at home.

> *Well tonight was a historical night for me. I went to the 31st Annual Grammy Awards. I was kissed [on the cheek] by Michael Hutchence, chatted with Sinéad O'Connor, and hugged by Anita Baker. Called Billy drunk off my ass from the INXS private party. This was quite probably the best night of my life... I know I sound like a complete groupie but hey, anyone would have felt that way. Also, Melissa Etheridge, Sinéad, Toni Childs, and Tracy Chapman performed and were absolutely spectacular... Oh yea, Alice Cooper watches* Married... *every week!*

I look back at these memories, people, and places, so gilded back then. Now I know that famous people are just humans going through the same shit we're all going through.

Life is messy no matter who is living it.

* * *

For all the compromises *Married... with Children* forced upon me with regard to my self-image, it was still my home away from home.

Creating a show took a week; we'd rehearse Monday through Thursday and then tape in front of a live audience each Friday. Most days I didn't have to be at work until 10 a.m., so my mom would bring my breakfast up to my room on a tray. She would make tofu scramble and a piece of toast and pour me a glass of pineapple juice. My mom would hand me the juice and say, "Let's wake up your mouth, Tini," and once my eyes had adjusted to the day, we'd sit on my bed and watch *The Brady Bunch* while I ate—we did that every morning for years, until I moved out.

Years we did that.

Years.

My mouth suitably energized, I'd head to rehearsal to join my other family. I was with that cast all week, and in effect I was raised by my mother, Ed O'Neill, Katey Sagal, and the rest of the adults on that cast and crew. In recent years, I've said about both Ed and Katey, "If people don't like me, you can blame them. And if people like me, you can blame them, too."

Ed was somewhat rough around the edges but incredibly funny. He's from Youngstown, Ohio, blue-collar, but he wasn't the hand-down-the-pants, Al Bundy kind of person. He was classy, not to mention a very smart, well-trained actor. He's still my dear friend, and I know that if I want to spend a couple of hours on the phone silently listening to a lovely human wax lyrical about every single thing under the sun, all I have to do is take his call, which of course I always do.

As for Katey Sagal, I'll never forget walking into the rehearsal studio for the first time. At the time, there were multiple spaces in one building where Columbia Pictures Television had all their rehearsal studios, for shows like *Who's the Boss?* and *Diff'rent Strokes* and *Married...* and many others.

I was fifteen years old and Katey was thirty, and I thought she was so hot. There she was, wearing the perfect pair of jeans, and there I was, a weird hippie girl with bells on my ankles. I wanted to look like Katey—tall with long thin legs and what I considered to be perfect boobs. I was enamored with her coolness. She'd put on those little heels, and she'd shimmy and do a Bette Midler walk across the stage and thereby create an indelible character—in fact, the show had four iconic characters (Al, Peggy, Bud, and Kelly) by the time it came to an end.

Offstage, Katey chain-smoked, and she originally smoked in the show, too, although that was eventually banned. The rehearsal studios were all jammed together in one building, and when we'd take our breaks, we'd head out to the hallway to throw a football around. Katey would light up, projecting an effortless cool. One day we were throwing the ball back and forth and the iconic Cloris Leachman came striding down the hallway—she was rehearsing a different show down the way. Cloris was a teeny, tiny little thing with a gorgeous ballet chest, shoulders back, poised. She walked with authority.

She took one look at me and announced, "You need to stop playing football and you need to stop smoking!"

In my head I thought, *Whatever.* But what I said out loud was, "I'm not smoking. Tell Katey. Don't talk to me about it."

Katey looked at Cloris and brushed her off.

"Yeah, yeah, okay..."

And that was that. Cloris left, and Katey kept smoking. Katey was a very tough, beautiful earth mother who had lived through so much stuff, and was just grateful to be alive. She wasn't about to have anyone tell her what to do, not even a legend like Cloris Leachman.

Our set had a wonderful atmosphere. It was fun; it was funny. These were the people I spent all day with every day. We were a bunch of broken people—beautiful, broken people, raising each other, regardless of our different ages. We were doing something no one had done since *All in the Family,* a show that had been centered on antiheroes, just as ours was.

Sarcastic was our "love language." We didn't have

deep conversations about life outright, but we *got* each other. Katey knew what I was going through outside the set. She didn't have to talk to me about it; she was just there. Ed would kick anyone's ass to protect me. I knew that they had my back. I didn't tell them very much about what I was going through—I didn't really tell anyone; I never have, until now, in these pages—but my family at *Married... with Children* just knew, in the way that families know. They knew to protect me without me even seeing it at the time.

I always remember this exchange from the show: Peggy asks Al, "What are you thinking?" Al says, "If I wanted you to know, I'd be talking." That sums up the show and the people and, honestly, my life.

But for a while I did feel a bit left out by everybody on *Married...* Back then, I didn't like snark, if you can believe it. I didn't cuss, except to myself in my diary. I didn't like bad things being said about other people, and I didn't like negative talk. Just as in any workplace, there would be gossip and people talking behind others' backs, but I would walk away when it started, like I was somehow above it. I was trying to uphold some kind of decorum, to eradicate the mess I felt inside. I think inadvertently I made them feel bad. (These days, I'm Mistress Snark.)

The truth was, I was in my own space, in my own head. I would write,

> *Wednesday, May 31, 1989*
> *Can't really tell how I'm feeling at this moment. A bit paranoid, a bit down, a bit giddy. But for some strange reason it all doesn't seem real. I'm alive, but right now I don't feel real. For the last 3 hours I've been fading into oblivion.*
>
> *Madness*
> *Pounding in my brain*
> *Why, I don't know*
> *Will you please hold me*
> *Because I'm insane.*
> *And I don't know what to do.*
> *How can I be happy one moment*
> *And feel like dying in the other?*

I'm sure everyone on set knew something was wrong. A demon had slipped into my life, a man I would only just survive.

SIX

NOSTRADAMUS

IN MY LATE TEENS, me and my mother and a friend of hers took a trip to Paris. When Mom and I headed back to the States, her friend stayed in France for another week and went to Père Lachaise to visit Jim Morrison's grave. She arrived to find a man lying across it while his friend took photographs. I suppose Morrison does that to people (though in my case, when I visited the grave, I knitted a scarf and drank an entire bottle of red wine. No cups). They all got to talking, and she called me a few days later to say that the guy on the grave was "the most amazing guy in the whole world. He's beautiful." When she came back to the States, she showed me pictures of him from magazines.

    A year or so later, I was heading to Hawaii while on break from *Married...*, and the same woman urged me to reach out to this guy. He was well-traveled, and she thought maybe he'd have some ideas about where I could go and what I could do. I called him, not thinking much of it. We stayed on the phone for hours. She had been right. He was engaging, even to my mind a bit eccentric. I continued to talk to him throughout my stay in Hawaii, and those conversations only deepened when I came back. My mom even told me that when I was away, he had been over to her house to see her. She urged me to meet him, too.

"Christina," she said, "he's the coolest guy. He's totally your type."

I asked him what his plans were for Mother's Day, and he bemoaned the fact that his mother was away. I didn't hesitate before inviting him to join us at our Mother's Day lunch.

That's where it all started. How I wish I'd never extended that invitation.

Years ago, there was a Moroccan restaurant on the corner of Sunset and Stanley called Dar Maghreb. Run by Pierre Dupar, a French chef of rotund proportions straight out of central casting or *Ratatouille*, Dar Maghreb was then the go-to place in Hollywood for special occasions, like a birthday or anniversary, or just when you felt like doing something different. The restaurant would proudly serve seven courses in its faux Middle Eastern setting, replete with colorful tiles, a fountain, and Arabic lettering on the walls. The waiters would bring mint tea to the table, which they'd pour from shoulder height to ensure that the correct amount of bubbles fizzed on the meniscus. All the while, belly dancers shimmied about, rattling their finger bells and wobbling their midriffs.

A perfect setting for Mother's Day lunch.

We drove to pick him up—it would be the first time I ever saw him in person. He slipped into the back seat, leaning forward to kiss me on both cheeks in the European fashion. I was immediately fascinated with him.

He held himself with confidence, something I found totally sexy. During the meal I kept waiting for my mother to go to the bathroom so we could be alone. He and I weren't even talking to each other very much, but there was an undeniable energy between us. When my mom finally stepped away, he moved to sit next to me and, without a word, picked up a strawberry from the table and held it to my mouth. Yes, he really did that—he fed me strawberries, and I thought it was sexy, intriguing, and a little bit creepy.

What can I say? I was still just a teenager.

He was intoxicating. No one had ever treated me like this. At that point in my life things were starting to finally feel like they were turning around. I was maturing out of childhood and into a place where I could make decisions for myself, and the deepest traumas, though stored away in my body, were nevertheless now a decade removed. *Married... with Children* was at its height. I was about to land my first "#1 on the call sheet" movie, *Don't Tell Mom the Babysitter's Dead*. I'd just moved out of my mother's house. Everything was new and exhilarating.

In the back of my mind, though, I knew I'd too often found myself in bad situations with men, situations that had caused pain and insecurity. These early loves hadn't been abusive, but they didn't seem to want the same level of commitment I needed. I wanted the ones who didn't want me. I was a romantic; I felt things very deeply. My diaries are filled with longing and hope and, I'm sorry to say, disappointment. I'd fall for someone, only to realize he didn't feel the same. My journals are littered with moments when men treated me less than kindly. Given that I already struggled with self-esteem, these "Does he love me?" relationships often made me feel even worse. Now, though, a handsome and confident man was feeding me strawberries in a Moroccan restaurant.

That was all it took.

Within a couple of days, we started hanging out, and from there it very quickly became a Thing. The relationship had the unstoppable momentum of a steam engine, our very own steamroller.

Only a few months later, I was referring to him as "wonderful" and "my boyfriend" in my diaries, yet even then—even then!—a small, too small voice in my head was trying to get a message to my better judgment. That very same month, when I was calling him my wonderful boyfriend, warning signs were already evident.

> *[He] and I are still together. We have problems sometimes, but not too major... I've been feeling pretty fucked lately. Just about my appearance, my life. What else is new? I find myself looking at old pictures, seeing my weight then, remembering my old beaus. I miss Billy and Sebastian sometimes. It's weird; I can't really explain it. I mean, I love [my boyfriend] very much. But I miss the others. Of course, Billy—I love him more than I could love any other man. I don't know why. He just means a great deal to me. And he and I will always know that one day we will marry each other. Of course, when no one wants us. But for now I'll be young and try to enjoy my life. Before my whole perfectness manifests.*

It seems so significant now, looking back, that not one month into the relationship I was a) feeling bad again about how I looked and b) fondly thinking of previous boyfriends.

Still, he was alluring in the way scumbags often are. He was tall and handsome, and then of course there were the strawberries. I've already said that I was tragically drawn to men about whom I should have known better, but I was all too comfortable thinking I could save or rehabilitate, or more often than not just pay the way of, the guys that I dated.

Within three months we were living together. By this time he was living in LA, and his lease was up. He either had to leave his apartment or move back to Paris, so he moved in. He was away working in France for a little while, and then when he got back, he asked me to marry him, as quickly as a red flag can be waved. I felt his talons sink into me a couple of weeks after he moved in.

I was madly in love with him, but something was always off. When I was filming *Don't Tell Mom the Babysitter's Dead,* I noticed he seemed unhappy about it, jealous that my time was being taken away from him. He would call up my mom and tell her, "I don't understand why she's not paying attention to me."

"Jesus!" my mom would say. "She's making a *movie.* She's the *star.* The whole ten-million-dollar film is on her shoulders. Let her do her thing."

Some days he'd come to set and pretend to be supportive, but I felt it was an act, almost like he was spying on me. Ladies, if a man starts to control your every move, get the fuck out. I didn't. One time he even said to me, "No one is ever going to love you the way I love you." Still, I steamrolled ahead.

At one point, I had to do a kissing scene, and I could feel his diabolical jealousy. I had seen this behavior before, when my mom was being controlled by men who didn't deserve her. But it was still early in the relationship, and I thought he was so beautiful, so I buried my fears.

Just like with *Married...*, I hadn't wanted to make *Don't Tell Mom the Babysitter's Dead* at first because it was a studio film. I wanted to do independent movies. I didn't want to "sell out." I thought the movie was cheesy, but then I thought everything was.

When it came out it was a huge flop, a flop that prevented me from getting jobs because right above the title was my name. It would eventually become one of the most quotable movies. I watched it recently and thought, *What a great and weird little movie.* All these years later, people are still saying, "I'm right on top of that." My character was an anti–teen idol, smoking cigarettes and cussing. I still remember insisting on wearing my green Doc Martens.

But she was just not what the world wanted at that

time, I think, and as a young woman in the public eye with painfully low self-esteem, I took it hard. He was the kind of boyfriend who could taste that on my skin, and he acted accordingly. Men like that don't tend to prey on strong women, and though I'd had a tough life already, I was sensitive and open and lacking in the kind of steel it would take me years to cultivate. I was a poet, for God's sake.

There were so many little things I felt he did to chip away at me, adding up to a relationship that left me in tatters. He didn't like my clothes, for a start, and would tell me what to wear instead. I could feel him get angry when I was eating too much, or even just when I was eating, which was hell for someone who already had a fucked-up relationship with food and her body. I was always terrified he'd turn up on set, too. To this day there is still a set of tire skid marks on the Highland exit of the 101 in Hollywood, left when I felt like he was trying to kill us as we got off the freeway one day. I've never been so scared in all my life.

I knew it wasn't right, but I was hooked. When something happened on my birthday that November, the small uneasy voice inside me became a scream. I should have fled then. But men like that have a way.

I was still living in the house behind the Country Store in Laurel Canyon, and one day I could hear him on the phone downstairs having a tempestuous argument with someone. When I went to see what was going on, he yelled, "You tell your fucking mother I don't want to fucking ever try to help her with anything ever again."

I was stunned. I asked him what had happened.

"They've been planning a surprise birthday party for you," he said, "and I was going to give her names of people who you really like, but they really don't care and they're really not involving me. They're doing it all themselves."

I was shocked by his childishness. You might think killing the surprise for me was bad enough—and for what sounded like completely ridiculous reasons—but what came next should have had me running to the hills.

I heard my mother's car pull in shortly after. She must have left her house as soon as he hung up on her. I walked outside to talk to her in the car.

"That fucking asshole!" she yelled. "There's something wrong with him."

She was sounding off when I noticed him bounding out of the house, down the driveway. I'd never seen this side of him before; I was terrified. Before I could stop him, I remember him thrusting half of his body through the open window of the car, screaming in my mother's face.

"Get your head out of your ass, you fucking bitch!" he was shouting.

In fear, she started to drive away. I saw him kick

the car. Again, I was speechless. What had happened? All I remember after that is the pit of devastation that lodged in my stomach. And yet I was still in the throes of obsession with him, so much so that at the subsequent birthday party, we all agreed that he would stay on one side of the club, and my mother would stay on the other.

I was desperate to keep the peace. I loved my mother more than I loved anyone, but I couldn't break his spell on me. I needed to please them both. I didn't want either of them to ruin the party for all my guests—friends who wanted to make me happy. If you look at the pictures of that birthday party, I seem very happy.

But as ever, my eyes aren't smiling.

This marked the true beginning of my excuses for him, trying to believe that everything would calm down and eventually be okay. In my heart I was thinking, *I can't lose him,* just as I had always thought about my mother, *I can't lose her.* He'd convinced me I'd never find anyone better than him, and I believed him.

Fear of abandonment was deep in my soul; my whole life, I had always felt that my mother was going to leave me. I feared she resented me for ruining her life. She was a great support, and a great love, but I was always afraid of upsetting her.

My mom hated him. She knew, she just *knew*. Of course she did. After what she'd been through with Joe Lala, she wanted to do anything she could to keep me away from the likes of this guy, but there was no telling me. She would say, "I know this guy is going to hurt you. Get the fuck away from him, Christina." She said she knew the look in his eyes, could feel this motherfucker's evil energy. As early as August 19, 1990, just a handful of months after the relationship started, I'd written,

> *My mom instills so much fear in me about him that it caused me to rummage through his things to see if he's some weirdo. But I found nothing but remnants of a very intense, confused, yet spiritual individual... I feel so empty. Sometimes I feel on the brink of desperate insanity. I'm afraid (today) to deal or talk to anyone from the outside world. Afraid, lonely, confused, bombarded, paranoid. All I can do is ask God to bring me back to the light. Feel it, taste it, inhale it, and digest it & drown in it.*

A few weeks later, I wrote this.

> [He] has gone to the Yucatan... I feel his main reason for going was because on Tuesday

he told my mother to get her head out of her fucking ass repeatedly. Not a good or a wise thing to do. She hates him now, as well as he hates her. For months I have been straining to bring them together. But that was the cause and Tuesday was the effect. It was my painful need to have peace. Now I am in hell. But I release them both. I will live this life for myself. Only for me. There is so much work for me to do on my own soul that any attempt to help others is falsely represented... If a goal is forced upon you, it only ends up working against it. So, yes, I desire for them to be at peace, but I will let the universe take care of that. This whole experience has left me physically chaotic. Hope the underlying effect that stress has on one will not result negatively in the future.

That last sentence chills me now, knowing all that is to come.

Yet even with the plain fact that my mother hated him, the progression of the relationship was swift, though I hardly sound deliriously in love.

We live together. But me? Well, I feel sort of lost... The one constant in my life is [him]. We have so much to learn about each other still. But it will happen in time. I've begun to really enjoy sex. Even though it's hard for me sometimes because of my body obsession. But all in all I suppose I'm happy...

...

Six months. We have been together for six fucking months. It's a miracle. There are so many hardships. But that's all part of it... He's crazy, I'm crazy. But we click so intensely where it is almost painful. I suppose a great deal of that pain is because love is such a rarity. Clawing to hold on. The jealousy. The rage. It all stems from love, passion, fear I suppose. My fear of being without him and at times with him. I've let go almost completely of all outside human contact. I don't want to be around anyone, only him. So unhealthy... We thrive on drama. And [he] and I deserve the Oscar. But I love him; I love his soul, so confused, like mine... Each day he becomes more and more beautiful to me. In my eyes he is the most beautiful man on Earth. It's funny, here I am writing all this and at the same time we're in a huge argument. I feel pretty mellow about it though. I can't let it get to me. I can't stomach it.

No more.

Bye for now.

* * *

My career was taking off in new ways. I smiled for the cameras while promoting *Married...* and *Don't Tell Mom the Babysitter's Dead* to hide everything that was happening in my relationship. These roles allowed me to move into a log cabin on Lookout Mountain Avenue by my early twenties. It was ten houses due west from where Joni Mitchell had lived two decades earlier. Maybe there I could feel "unfettered and alive."

That log cabin was the most beautiful property I could have imagined, with every kind of fruit tree thriving on the grounds: apples, oranges, tangerines, pears. There were avocados and grapes and thirty or forty rosebushes of every variety and color. I could live off the fruit and sometimes did, lasting a whole week or longer on the windfall of my yard.

When I bought it, it had already been christened Rogues Retreat. I kept the name, and the original old wooden sign with the name etched on it. There was wisteria that had grown around and into and on top of a pergola — it looked as though the pergola had disappeared and this powerful wisteria vine was magically suspended in the air. Out back we had a fireplace and picnic tables. To get to the house itself required navigating nearly eighty stairs up from street level — I stole a shopping cart from somewhere so that when I got groceries, I'd be able to get them up the initial ramp, though that would still leave me with a hefty climb. I'd drag ten or fifteen bags all the way up to the kitchen so I would have supplies for the night's festivities — the house was always full.

Everyone came up and hung out at Rogues Retreat. I had a yard, which was a new experience for me and for all my Canyon friends. The idyllic childhoods we'd all missed were now played out as adults in the confines of my house and garden. Sometimes we'd make a slip-and-slide and hoot and holler all the way down to the edge of the property. Or I would put together an Easter egg hunt, stashing a hundred bucks in the golden egg, and watch as my friends knocked each other over and rolled all the way down the hill to try to score the cash. We were an out-of-control gang of young adults screaming and fighting and shoving each other and screeching with laughter. It was magical.

I'm sure the neighbors hated us. We didn't give a shit.

Inside the house I'd built a dance studio — of course I had — and installed a huge, heavy four-poster in the main bedroom. The house boasted its original stone fireplace and a little cubby for an old-timey phone, all built in 1918, when it was erected. There was a huge living room — the biggest I'd ever seen, I thought, after living in the 750-square-foot house up the hill — with an expansive bay window, and high ceilings stretching up to the loft area. I had a pool table just like at my grandparents' place in Indiana, only mine was in my dining room. The kitchen in the log cabin was tiny, I suppose, but we spent most of our time outside barbecuing anyway. During the Northridge earthquake in 1994, my huge four-poster bed slid right across the room. One lamp fell and shattered, and a single brick flew off my fireplace, but other than that, those houses in the Canyon were sturdily built, especially my cherished log cabin. The place escaped any real or lasting damage.

We were young and stupid, a bunch of idiot dickheads, but we threw great parties. I was home base, and I loved every second of it. We would run around that property like it was Lord of the fucking Flies, doing whatever we wanted to do.

It was a haven, for me and all my friends, even as I felt my boyfriend's claws sink in deeper.

When I try to understand that relationship now, the only way I can do so is by excavating my early childhood. My father had left when I was a baby; my mother had brought Lala into our lives, and had occasionally left me alone for hours, too. I don't suppose it takes a highly trained psychologist to see the abandonment issues—the truth was, I never felt like I was truly taken care of. So when it seemed like someone was into me, really cared about me, well, I quickly bought in, even if it turned out to be bullshit. I wanted to believe that I was everything to someone so badly. I needed that validation because I didn't really value myself at all. If a man appeared to love me, and passionately love me at that, I never knew if that was the last time this was going to happen, so I put up with everything else.

I hated myself; I thought I was ugly and fat and stupid and uncool. This guy offered me protection and what I thought was love. I was desperate to have that, and it registered as some fun house version of happiness. I totally adored him.

I hadn't had many lovers by then — I would describe myself as "still kind of a virgin" at the time, or at least inexperienced and naive. We had waited a month to sleep together, and when we did, our bliss had kept us up until six in the morning (well, coupled with the first and last time I took ecstasy). With the dawn breaking, he headed down to the 7-Eleven on Sunset and bought champagne and orange juice, and we sat outside on the swing, drinking and basking in the love we'd shared.

After that initial bliss, we never really had the romance of going on real dates — we'd just hang out in the house. I introduced him to John Frusciante and the rest of that Chili Pepper crowd I knew. John thought he was cool, but it didn't stick. We didn't become one big happy house with two cats in the yard. Pretty quickly, I was isolating, blocking out my friends, closing off the circle of people around me, staying in when previously I'd been out and about in Los Angeles.

I just became the girlfriend. I felt like this man took control of my friend group, talking poisonously about them to me, isolating me from them. I had no idea what was happening behind the scenes. I just thought I'd found the love of my life, and we were wrapped up in our own world. Retrospectively, I can see that familiar pattern of cutting out friends so that someone can be the number one. It was always the same thing: "No one loves you the way I love you."

I know now that a lot of people hated him and wanted me away from him. But people so often don't do anything about it, and so the dark and painful vortex kept spinning tighter and tighter.

It wasn't just my mother and peers who had reservations about this guy: the cast of *Married...with Children* felt he was trouble, too.

In the spring of 1992, as part of the upcoming season 6 it was decided that *Married...with Children* would decamp to England to film a three-episode story set in the UK. I have no idea why anyone thought it made sense to have the Bundys in Britain—I'm not sure I can think of a less likely combination than raw Bundy bawdiness in the land of abject politeness—but there we were, filming at all the clichéd locations, like Buckingham Palace and Harrods and Hyde Park Corner and Heathrow Airport, as well as way out in the Kent countryside.

My boyfriend came with us, and my colleagues' disdain became clear pretty quickly. In fact, I thought Ed O'Neill was going to punch that motherfucker out, he hated him so much. If I was ever to ask Ed about him, I'm sure I'd be met with a two-hour monologue of loathing even today.

I remember him causing trouble from the very beginning. I couldn't leave the house in tight clothes. I always had to wear a bra. I wasn't allowed to wear form-fitting clothes on the show anymore. I had to change my whole wardrobe. The unhappiness made me gain weight, which he also hated. I was living in hell.

On the plane back from Europe, I ate two pieces of shrimp and some cocktail sauce. I remember the exact number—that's how neurotic I was. I ate them in the bathroom so my boyfriend wouldn't see, but he clocked my empty plate when I got back to my seat anyway.

"Why are you eating so much?" he said.

After that I started hiding food when I ate. I was a TV star, and a movie star, a young woman who regularly appeared on talk shows and red carpets and awards shows, confidently striding through life, looking everyone in the eye. In private, I was telling myself I'd never find anyone like him, never find anyone who was going to love me as much as he loved me. I thought, *I'm not good enough, not attractive enough to have anyone or have anything that I deserve.* As my fame grew, my self-esteem shrank—I wished someone would notice, but when you're a celebrity, your life looks like a cakewalk. My sad eyes were crying, but no one could see.

I felt his controlling nature worsen. During one altercation, I fell against my car in my garage. The argument continued out onto the gravel path up to the steps that led to my house. I think he pushed me, and I fell on the path, where I rubbed my face on the stones until I bled. I did so because I was so desperate to be seen, for someone—especially someone I worked with—to notice, so I didn't have to tell anyone with words.

I wanted to be saved.

In the end, I was.

In 1992, when Bill Clinton was running for president, Richard Dreyfuss had invited a bunch of actors to his house to establish a get-out-the-vote push, and he included me because he thought I represented the youthful side of Hollywood. Richard handed us huge stacks of register-to-vote paperwork and asked me to take it to places where "the young people" congregated.

I had bought Rogues Retreat from the people who owned a spot in Hollywood called the Sunset Social

Club, and I asked them if I could bring the registration forms to the club.

Before I headed to the club, my boyfriend and I had a terrible fight. It had ended, like so many others, with him berating me, but I can't even remember what it was about now — that's how routine it had become. When I arrived, I couldn't shove it down. The owners could see that I had tears in my eyes and that I was shaking.

The owner took one look at me and said, "You are of no use right now." It was honestly nice to be seen, for once to be let off the hook. He gestured over to a table with a group of young women. "Go sit with them." When I sat down, I could hardly breathe, but these women who I didn't know at all rallied around me. They ordered me vodka gimlets — my grandmother's drink. I loved them. At that table was Shannon, Carolyn, Tommi, and China.

Those women are still my best friends to this day. They're the only people I will let in my bedroom and the only people I will let lie in my bed next to me. They saw me at my worst and rallied around a stranger. They were punk rock bitches, and they weren't going to let a man fuck with them or anyone they cared about. It was a strength and resolve I desperately needed at the time. I still think of how random that moment was, how easily it could have never happened.

There is something special about the way women see each other. The way we immediately had a shared language, especially when it came to understanding what I was going through with my boyfriend at the time.

Shannon is gorgeous, stupidly gorgeous, and deliciously mean when she needs to be. She was perfectly comfortable kicking people out of bars if they pissed her off—she is a punk rock skater girl at heart. She's been through a lot, seen a lot, done a lot. She has beautiful kids. Really smart, really eccentric, interesting, brilliant children, highly politically charged. She's my friend who posts everything about this march and that march, fuck the government, fuck the patriarchy. She wants to change the world. And I love that about her. I'm a turtle. I like to go into my shell. But Shannon is intense, and so funny. We've done everything together, from traveling to taking French lessons to getting kicked out of Formosa Café together. She's my rock.

And then there's Carolyn. She grew up with Shannon in San Jose and was even a competitive skateboarder at one point. Throughout our lives, our paths have crossed and uncrossed. She went off to have kids before any of us did, while I was working so much, but when I got sick, Carolyn was there. And now Carolyn's with me almost every week.

Tommi, also part of what became the Viper Room

club, is what I call lusciously eccentric. She's married to magician Rob Zabrecky, a fantastic musician and former lead singer of Possum Dixon. When Rob started doing magic, he and Tommi would take a break in the middle of the show and tap-dance onstage. They've been together for almost thirty years now and they're perfect together, both beautifully weird and loving and kind.

China—who happens to be Grace Slick's daughter—is the funny, raw, unapologetic, chain-smoking heart of our group. These days she's a sober Christian pastor, but whenever I see her, she'll still sit and just be China.

Along with Pharel from my childhood, these beautiful women are scrappy as fuck, righteous as fuck. They are my girls, my tribe. They would do anything for me. All my friends are wonderfully strange and beautiful and kind, but they will also beat up someone for you. We've all changed across the years—become mothers, or taken the cloth, or whatever—but whenever we get together, it's like we are still the same group we were way back when we first met, back in that club drinking vodka gimlets. Except these days when we meet, I'm not crying. I'm swearing and laughing. They gave me their energy.

By the end of that first night, I was a little buzzed and had gotten rid of my huge stack of registrations, and then that Clinton guy won. I like to think his victory was entirely down to me.

These girls saved me, but not all in one night. My relationship with this man went on, but they sparked something inside me.

I had to be my own savior. I always fought back, I always physically struggled, but sometimes I feared that was so that he would hurt me more. I think part of me wanted him to hurt me. I wanted him to beat the shit out of me. I wanted him to beat my face up. It took me years to understand why—and then I realized it was because I wanted help. Just like when I was younger and I would take pills or cut myself, I wanted someone to say, "My god, look what he's done to you. We'll get rid of him for you." I didn't know how to do it myself—in fact, it wasn't even an option. We must have broken up eight or nine times throughout the relationship, and each time he'd guilt and woo himself back into my life, saying things like "You need to give me five thousand dollars because you're making me homeless."

On one of the occasions when we broke up, he left and went to San Francisco. When he called me a few days later, I faked trying to kill myself, faked that I was stabbing myself—this is how ridiculous the whole situation was. I wanted him to feel as bad as I felt. I would do anything to try to make him feel guilty for what he'd been doing to me.

But instead of showing guilt, or concern, or God forbid realizing the damage he was doing, he drove all the way down from San Francisco and showed up in my house. I woke up to him looming over me, like he'd caught me in a lie, which I suppose he had.

On and on I stayed with him, with a constant and futile determination to turn it around, turn him around.

In late April 1991, I fell pregnant. I want to turn away from what happened, but it's all recorded in my diary. There are moments in my life that are too painful to force into narrative or meaning, so I'll let my voice from back then speak.

> *Well, yesterday I found out I was 6½ weeks pregnant. Too many emotions are filling my soul. I love this being. Anyway, two days before I found out, I got into a car accident on the way to the gynecologist. My car didn't survive, but luckily, I did. I knew I was pregnant. I couldn't understand why even*

though I was watching my eating I still felt fat. I couldn't understand why sex made me sick and I cried at the drop of a hat. Now I know. I always felt that if I ever got pregnant when I knew it was the wrong time, I wouldn't have any problem having an abortion. "Oh, whatever, it isn't even a baby yet." That's bullshit. This creature is incredible. It makes me feel whole, safe... My boyfriend said I was a disgusting, self-obsessed, eating-disordered fat pig today (not in so many words). That opened my eyes a great deal... I don't really understand my relationship anymore. It isn't good. Sometimes I don't think it's worth it. It all started to get heavy when we moved into the new house, which, by the way, is fabulously, incredibly beautiful. Maybe I just want to enjoy it on my own. Maybe I want to have whoever over whenever I want... I feel I have lost myself somewhere, and I can't find her for the life of me.

Only days later, my diary takes a brutal turn.

I'm fucking pregnant and I'm killing my child on Thursday. I'm thinking where the fuck can

You with the Sad Eyes

> *I go to recuperate from murder... His family will hate me when they find out that I killed their family member because they don't believe in it. But I can't have this baby because I have work to do to entertain this fucking world. Besides, I can't... now.*

It breaks my heart, reading these pages. On June 9, I wrote a poem to my child, convinced it was a baby girl. I have no actual proof, but that doesn't matter: to this day, I *know*.

> *Hello little thing.*
> *I feel you every moment of my day*
> *Such a tiny existence*
> *Such an immense effect you have*
> *...*
> *You are a miracle*
> *A tiny-handed miracle*
> *I love you.*
> *But you know your fate.*
> *It is not your time.*
> *I know you didn't make the decision.*
> *But it can't be your time.*
> *You will live on, though...*
> *You will live through another.*
> *...*

*I hope you will forgive me.
But I want you to know how you've
changed me.
You've opened my eyes.
You're letting me know something is
more important than myself.
But Mommy can't be with you right
now.
But know she loves you
More than any other miracle.
And know that when it's your time
It will be your time.*

There is a page with various sentences blacked out, like a redacted government report, written the night before I had my abortion. I was afraid, terrified my boyfriend would read what I had written about him.

Wednesday, June 12, 1991
    Tomorrow is the day. Yes, pain and all the other emotions are pummeling my soul. But that is a whole other chapter. My main frustration/ ▇▇▇▇ *etc. is basically geared towards my "relationship," or whatever the fuck you want to call it. Maybe it's the pregnancy, I don't know, but at this moment in time* ▇▇▇▇ *The sick part that I don't understand is that I love*

him. But right now ▮▮▮▮ I ▮▮▮▮ I do not ▮▮▮▮ I ▮▮▮▮ I don't want to ▮▮▮▮ I do not want to try to work it out... Right now, all I want is silence, I want my life back, my privacy, my love for myself. But it is virtually impossible when one continues to put you down. Now, I'm sure I'm imagining most of it...

Then it was done.

Thursday, June 13, 1991
   Well, it's over. I feel pretty okay. Just kind of woozy. That gives me no time to realize what I have done. Which is most likely the best right now. I was looking over what I'd written yesterday and just have to laugh. My emotions were extremely warped (I really don't feel that way). Honestly, I think when you're pregnant you tend to feel that way about the male figure in your life... My life is pretty wild. I could seriously write a book. I guess this kind of is.

*   *   *

When you're at the bottom of a well, you can often see light, way up there, a distant sky of hope, but that doesn't mean you can easily climb out.

It's clear from my journals that I was struggling not only with him, but with myself. This is also one of the first times that my diary sounds prescient — it's almost as if I could see a future in which the bill for all the guilt and unhappiness and trauma would be paid by my body. Maybe it's just the long hours I have been spending on my bed thinking about my illness, but in reading these words from more than three decades ago, I find that I suffer a kind of concussive awareness of the future impact of all these dark events from my early life.

> *Saturday, September 14, 1991*
> *Change is needed desperately or else I will fucking shoot myself because I'm so tired of living a depressed fucked-up lie. Yeah I've had some good, sure, but mostly plain torture to myself. Mainly by not speaking my mind. Standing up for my honest immediate feeling. That word "sorry" sucks. It's bullshit. I've been wrong. Maybe I've caused it. Maybe I fucked up. Didn't handle it correctly. But I can't be sorry. I can't feel guilty. Guilt is not an emotion, it's a disease. A pathetic life-altering and*

in the long run fatal disease. A slow-process disease... It begins in the brain, then spreads the illness throughout the entire body until not only does the mind shut off, but the body as well.

"*A slow-process disease... It begins in the brain.*" It seems poetically fitting, and devastating, that I now suffer from a condition in which my body's very immune system—the thing that should save me from harm—has turned in on itself and attacked the myelin that protects my nervous system. I spent so much of my life racked with guilt that it's no surprise to me that it felt like a disease when I was younger, and has, in some ways, felt like the driving force of a disease I suffer now that I'm older.

"*Long run fatal...*" There is no cure for MS, and no one knows why anyone gets it, so my contention in this diary entry from 1991 makes just as much sense as anything. I didn't know back then that one day I would be mostly bedbound with MS, but I did know that something very dangerous was happening inside my soul, something that might one day *shut off my body*.

These journals I turn to read like prophecies as much as a historical record. Who knew I was the Nostradamus of Laurel Canyon?

* * *

Things began to crack. I started writing about what it would be like to be single, and started expressing self-awareness of his direct impact on my deteriorating confidence. His sway and the love I thought I felt kept me coming back, but I see the early signs of escape. It was torture, an internal battle every day. I would think, *Here's somebody who I hate more than anyone on the planet. But he gives me flowers. But I hate him. But he tells me he loves me. But I hate him.* Over and over and over.

> *Sunday, November 10, 1991*
> *A scenario repeated one too many times. [He] is angry and had barely spoken a word in two days. I acted wrongly on Friday, made, once again, an ass of myself. Now I must live in this punishment. I don't know where to turn. I'm constantly "fucking up," but with what? Who knows why what where. I used to be confident in knowing I was a good person, despite my neuroses. But since I've been in this relationship, my confidence in myself has deteriorated. I can't seem to please him, no matter what I do. I sabotage everything. My motives are right, but as he always says, I'm*

only 19 and acting accordingly. Funny how most 19-year-olds own a house, keep it together, cook for their boyfriend, have a job, are responsible? But I suppose I'm just a fucking kid, right? Lived through life and still managed to have a fucking sense of humor. A tolerable temper. Gee!! But there are more-together, wiser ones out there... When someone is always telling you what's wrong w/ you and not balancing out w/ what is good then it is hard to be able to stand back and evaluate. Just getting pushed down further into the depths of depression. So what do you do? Have space? What space? I am on a constant, never a chance to breathe... Please God lead me to the bliss I once felt, the freedom I once felt. Been a long time since I felt that.

SEVEN

THE ORANGE CURTAINS

It is Christmas, 1991. I invite my boyfriend to Indiana with me. I can't stand the fact that he is going to be alone. It broke my heart, even though he is also breaking my heart. I bought his ticket, as usual, the caretaker. Of course he ran into problems while traveling, though everything was a problem for him. I couldn't do anything right. I'd discovered just how meticulous about things he was, how anal about the way he wanted things to be. His laundry had to be folded a certain way, and I cooked for him every day after I got home from work. Even when I bought him a plane ticket, it was my fault the flight didn't go exactly the right way, like the relationship's energy had seeped out into the world.

We are at my grandmother's house for Christmas. My mom is with me, and Aunt Janet has come as usual, too. My mom has been very wary about me inviting my boyfriend, but I wanted him to see this Indiana Christmas because it was so important to me. His luggage has gone who knows where, and everyone has gone to sleep by the time he lands in South Bend after a screwed-up layover in Chicago. When I get to the airport in my cab, I can see him through the window, lying on the ground with a small backpack and his flute and his saxophone and his 16-millimeter camera. He always called himself a musician, but I've heard cats getting killed by coyotes in the Canyon and that sounded better.

Shit, I think, *there's going to be a fight.* I can just tell by his body language that he is pissed. Sure enough, when I go in to get him, he blames the entire travel fiasco on me, as though the airlines and the Midwest weather patterns are in my control. He yells at me in front of the cab driver all the way to my grandmother's—he loves to berate me in front of people, loves to make me look like an asshole, and there I am, a captive audience for his abuse. The cab driver keeps looking ahead at the sleet falling, though I think he recognizes me. I feel the irony of my fame growing as this man is dragging me down, making me feel like a worthless nobody. I want the world to stop. I want the sleet to become snow and bury us all.

By the time we get to the house, he has turned into a charmer, his anger having blown through like the storm outside, all smiles and warmth the next morning over coffee with my family.

The house is, as ever, lovely for Christmas. My boyfriend loves the painted photographs my grandfather once created and was so impressed by the artwork he found in the basement that he even starts to suggest he is the reincarnation of my grandfather, which when I think of it now is nothing short of unhinged.

Still, I can't see him for who he is. To do that, I'd have to see myself more clearly, and when I look at myself, all I see are flaws. Not only do I have sad eyes, I have eyes that are warped, the picture blurred, the perspective askew.

Christmas Eve is also my uncle Harry's birthday, and we all go out to dinner and have a lovely, sweet time. When we get back from the restaurant, we gather around to watch a video compilation of films my grandfather made throughout his life, from age nineteen until just before he died. They are cool home videos, if not exactly earth-shattering—the usual fare of an ordinary life in an ordinary town. They mean something to us, though, but likely little to anyone outside the family.

Halfway through the screening, however, my boyfriend starts extolling my grandfather as a visionary and an artist, when the truth is that he was abusive, once hitting my grandmother so hard she lost her hearing in one ear. My boyfriend raises his voice, wanting his praise to be heard above the talking and laughing as the video plays. No one's being rude; it's just the way of a family.

But I can see my boyfriend getting frustrated; it appears he is the only person here who has the full measure of my grandfather, and we're just heathens and Neanderthals for not giving him his full due. Eventually, he goes upstairs and starts fiddling with his own 16-millimeter camera in the bedroom in the dark. When I go up to see what he's doing, I find him crying. And then from the darkness he explodes.

"Nobody understands about this man," he wails. "Nobody understands what he was. And your family is just yakking all over it!"

I am flabbergasted. This kind of unhinged, not to mention over-the-top, reaction is beyond anything I'd seen so far, and that's saying something. I stare at him as the hallway light reflects eerily on his tortured face, and then I finally say it.

"You are such an asshole." And I close the door on him.

Thinking that was the end of it, and that he'll probably apologize for his outburst once he's calmed down, I go to the bathroom next door and pull down my pants to pee. As I'm sitting there, I hear heavy footsteps and tense up.

He comes barging in, grabs me around the neck, and drags me by my legs across the hallway, back to the bedroom, where the lights are still out. There he pins me to the bed, my pants still around my ankles. He's livid, lost to his anger, shaking with rage, fuming and foaming as though his life is on the line.

"What did you call me? The fuck did you call me?" He's really yelling now. And I realize it's not his life on the line: it's mine.

From downstairs I hear my mother's voice.

"Hey, what's going on up there?"

I whisper in his ear as he keeps pinning me down, "Please, whatever you do, just pretend we're making out. I don't want them to see this."

My mother, not getting an answer, comes upstairs, strides into the bedroom, turns on the light, and is horrified by what she sees.

"You tell your fucking daughter to shut her fucking mouth," he says. "She's being completely out of line." With that he unpins me and storms downstairs.

My mother, who has seen all too much of this kind of thing in her own life, is shaking.

"What is going on?" she says.

I sit up, pull up my pants, and try to seem okay.

"Nothing, nothing, nothing, nothing," I say, though the fear in my eyes and my shaking hands tell a different story.

While he's on his way down to the basement, my grandmother notices the rage in his eyes and becomes terrified herself, because she's seen that look before on her own husband's face, just as my mother has seen it on Lala's. Both my mother and my aunt go try to calm the guy down, but when my mother tells Janet what she's seen upstairs, that is it.

"You son of a bitch," Janet says, storming upstairs to call the cops.

There has seldom ever been a cop car on Victoria Street. When they arrive, the neighbors' jungle telegraph brings folks out of their houses to see what is up. The cops step in, almost apologetically, and find the guy sitting glumly downstairs. I'm asked if I want to press charges; I barely look up from the ground when I say no.

"Everything's fine, everything's fine, everything's fine," I say a little too eagerly. Who knows why we don't have him hauled away, but we don't—we women were all victims of abuse in one form or another, and it can be almost impossible to break out of a cycle like that, especially in a moment of great duress like this.

One of the cops speaks up. "Well, if we have any more disturbances from this house, we're going to arrest you, young man."

"Fine," he says, "then fucking arrest me..."

I'm terrified at this point, but I manage to haltingly tell him to shut up. My mom is basically holding me up; I can barely put a sentence together because of the coruscating feelings inside me.

Part of me wants him to get arrested so he can get

the hell out of my life finally, but part of me doesn't... because I love him and because, as ever, I feel like I can save him, and by saving him, save myself from all the dark feelings I carry. He was creative and interesting. He looked at life through a different lens, and I wanted that. In my mind, actors were *less* interesting — I liked the guy who looked at others' trash and saw the beauty. I thought that going against the grain of what was expected of me was where I would find comfort. I was still just a kid rebelling against my surroundings.

Once the cops leave, my aunt Janet takes over.

"Your grandmother's upstairs and her face is bright red," she says to me. "She's terrified. And you know she has a heart condition. I want him out of here. Now."

It is decided that he'll be taken to a motel that night. He reluctantly goes to get his stuff, and then we walk out of the house, he and I and my mother.

But I've seen this movie before. When he's angry, even his walk fumes. When I heard him coming toward the bathroom a few minutes earlier, I knew, I just knew, that it wasn't going to end well. His footfall would shake the ground, he would almost stomp, his eyes seemed to fill with rage and evil. It was a malevolence I'd never witnessed in any other human being; when he lost it, it seemed like he turned into a monster.

This is the version of him that walks out of my grandmother's house and gets into the back of the car with me as my mother gets into the driver's seat that

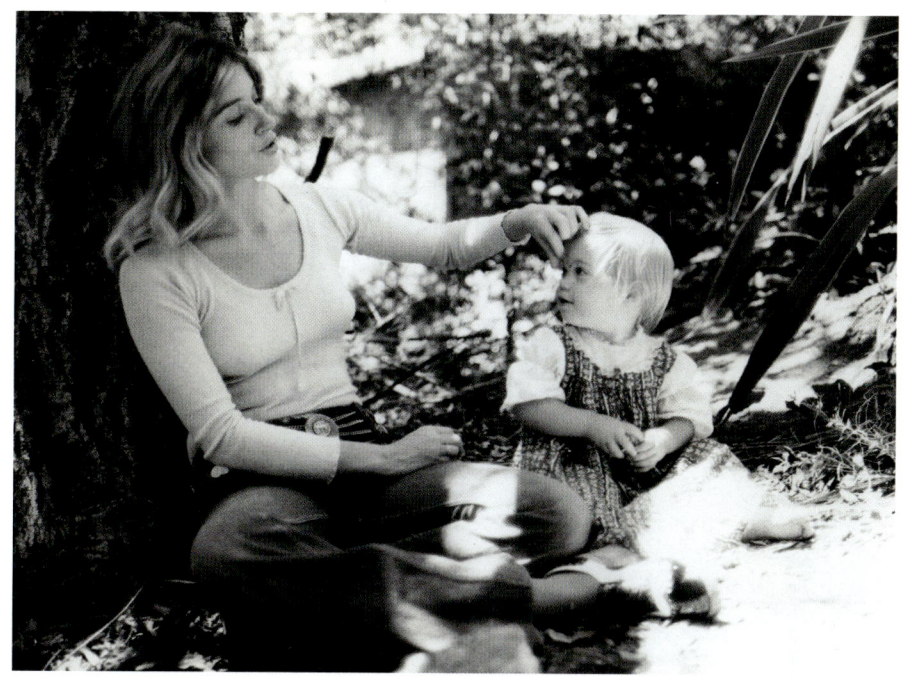

My beautiful mother.

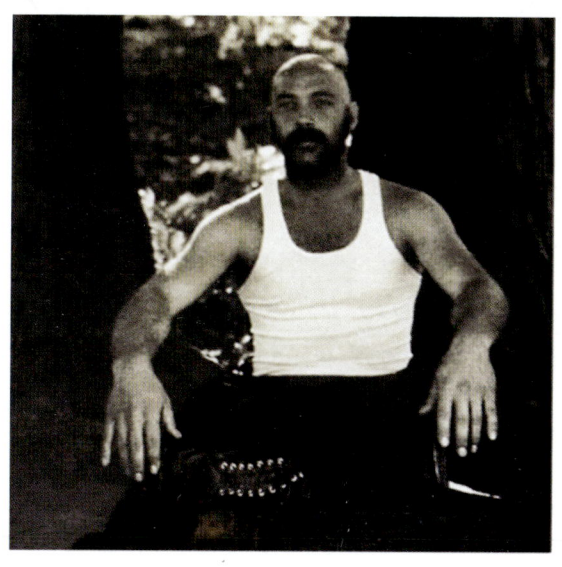

My dad in Big Sur.

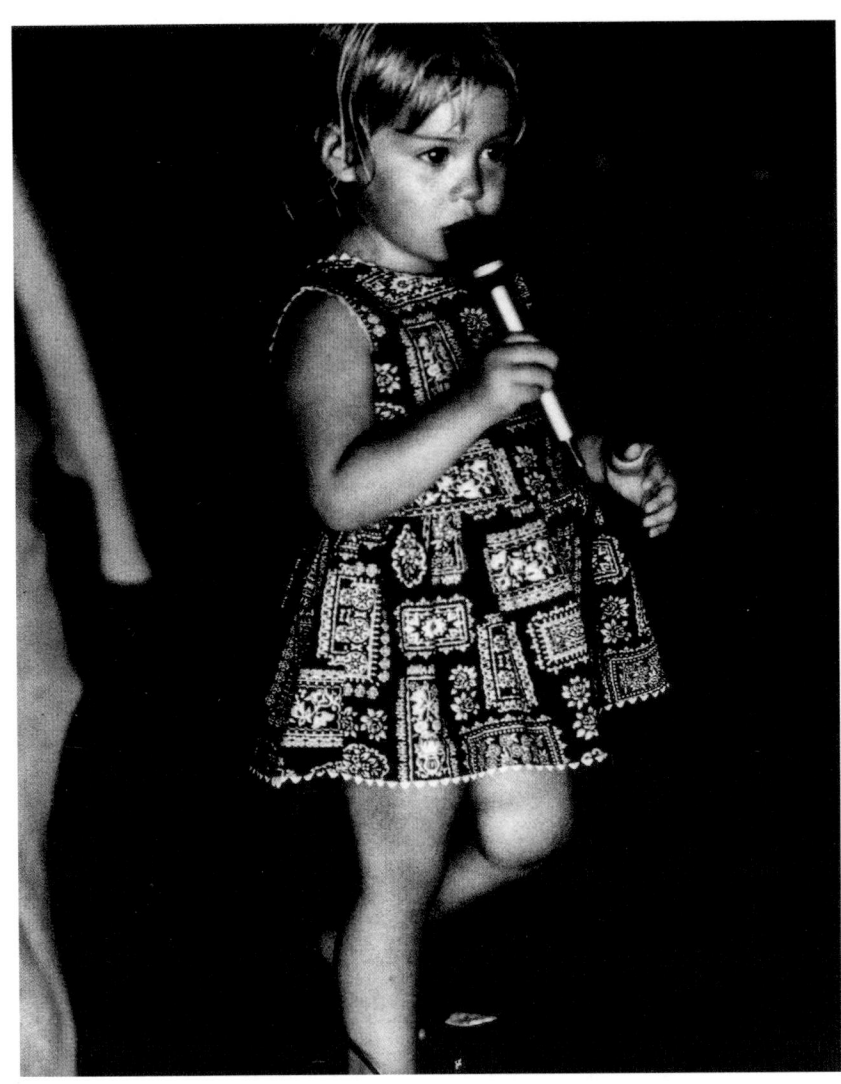

Singing to my parents' rock and roll friends.

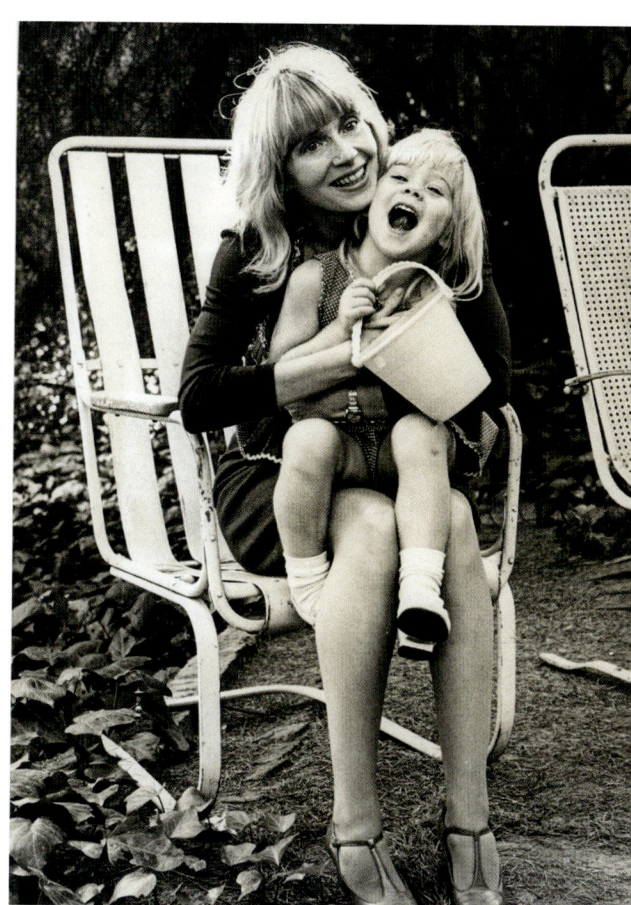

There was joy.

I hated being a Brownie.
I got kicked out for cussing.

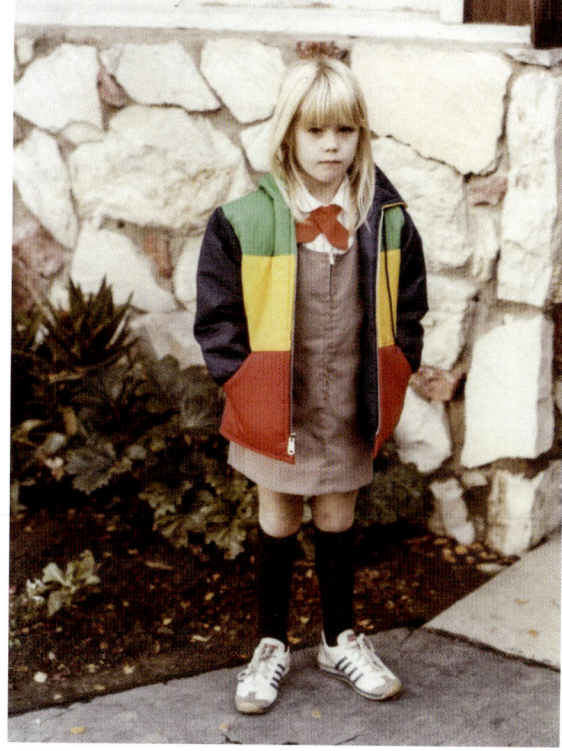

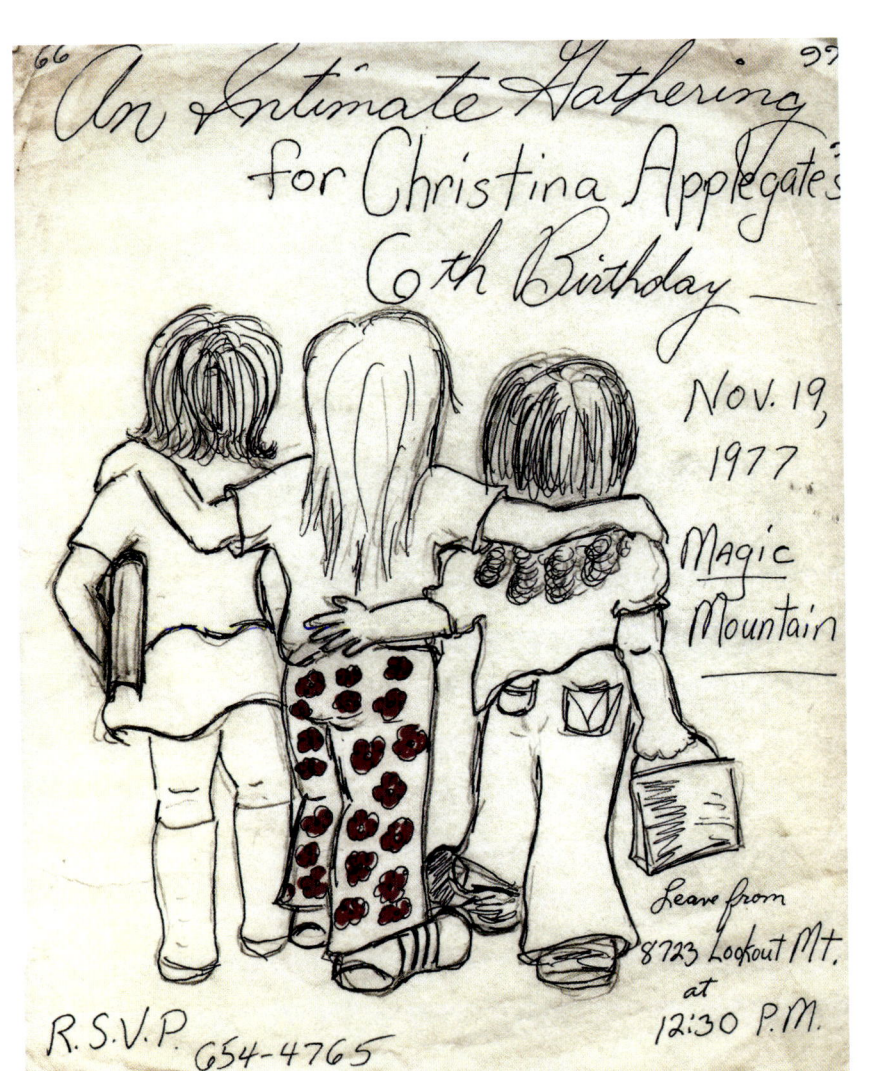

My mom drew handmade invites for every single birthday I had when I was little.

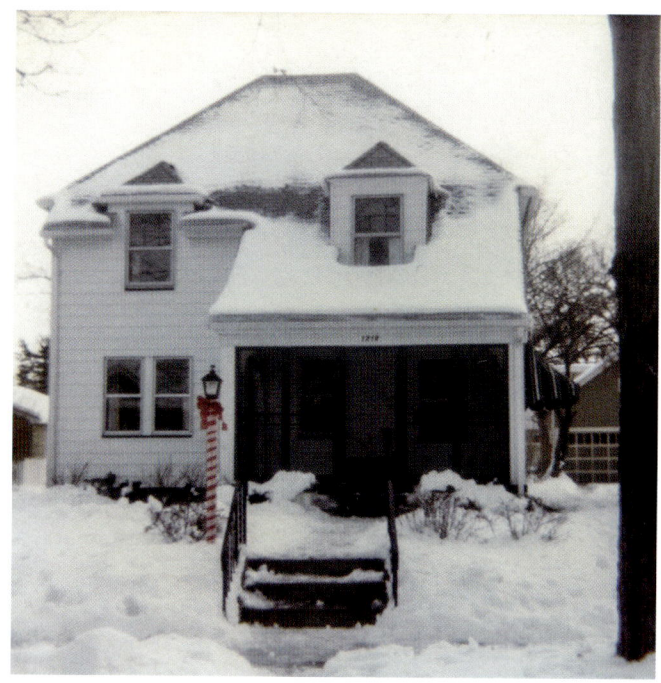

My grandmother's house in South Bend, Indiana. I loved that house. It was my favorite place to be. Merry Christmas.

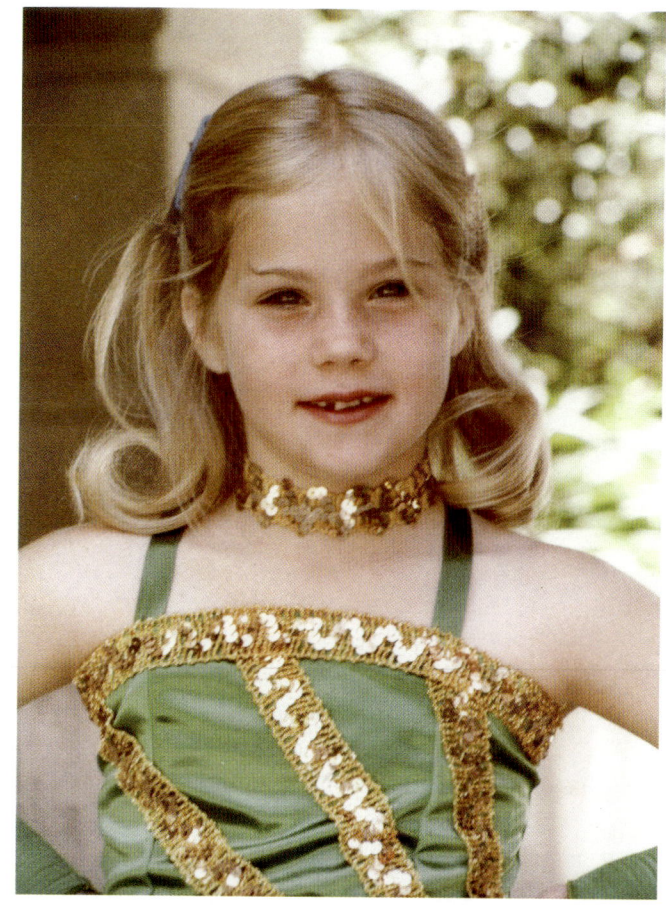

Me at a dance recital. My mom made the costume. I always loved to dance.

December 13, 1984

~~JANUARY 22~~ December 13, 1984

Know what? Michael and his friend Jacob came over to my house. Niki and Mariah were both over too. You'll not believe who I'm going out with. Fitz. Can you believe that? He might be going to my grandma's with me for a whole week! That will be the coolest xmas I'll ever have. My God. Breakfast, Lunch, and dinner spent with him. I love him so much. I'm sick now. I have strep. Niki likes Mike Farrell. Natalie is going out with him. Niki doesn't know that. I want to tell her but I cant. My life is so good. Oh! My mom caught me smoking in front of the Trax. So now I quit. I got in so much trouble! Gotta go

Love me.

Love, thirteen-year-old me.

January 12, 1985

Know what? Michael went with me to grandma's. I hate him. He is the biggest asshole in the whole world. I'm gonna break up with him tonight. Well, here is some other juicy news! Niki is going out with Alex. Which I think is great. And also I did another episode on "Charles in Charge" this week. It was great. I get the best feeling when I'm on that Lot. It's great. I'm so tired because of this week. I haven't been in school for a long time. I was sick a week, vacation for 2 weeks, then a week of "Charles". I'm scared to go back. I think I might like Zach! don't tell anyone! Love me

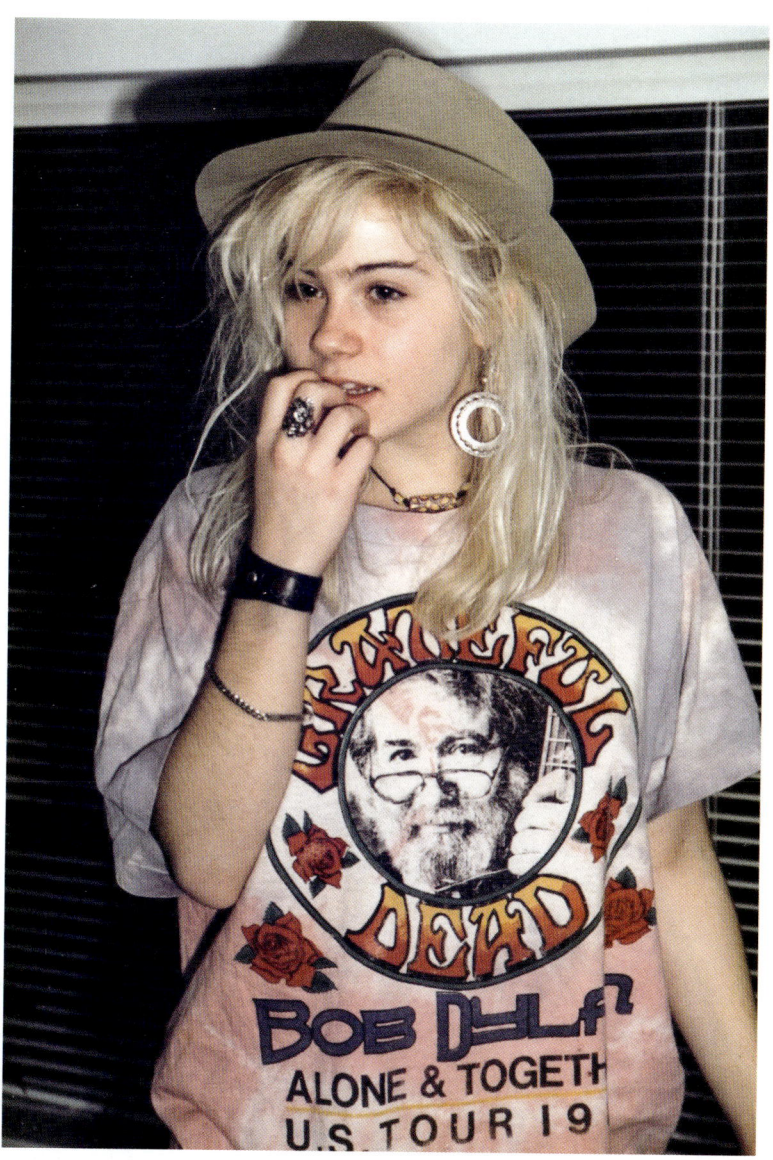

My unique teen fashion sense. What was I doing?

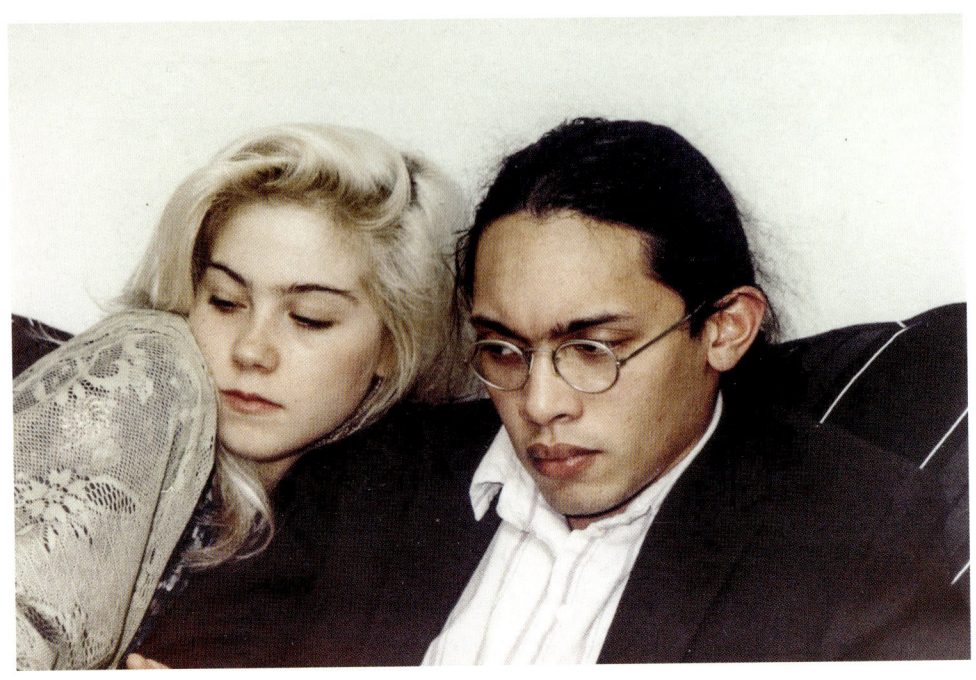

My dear friend Sam.

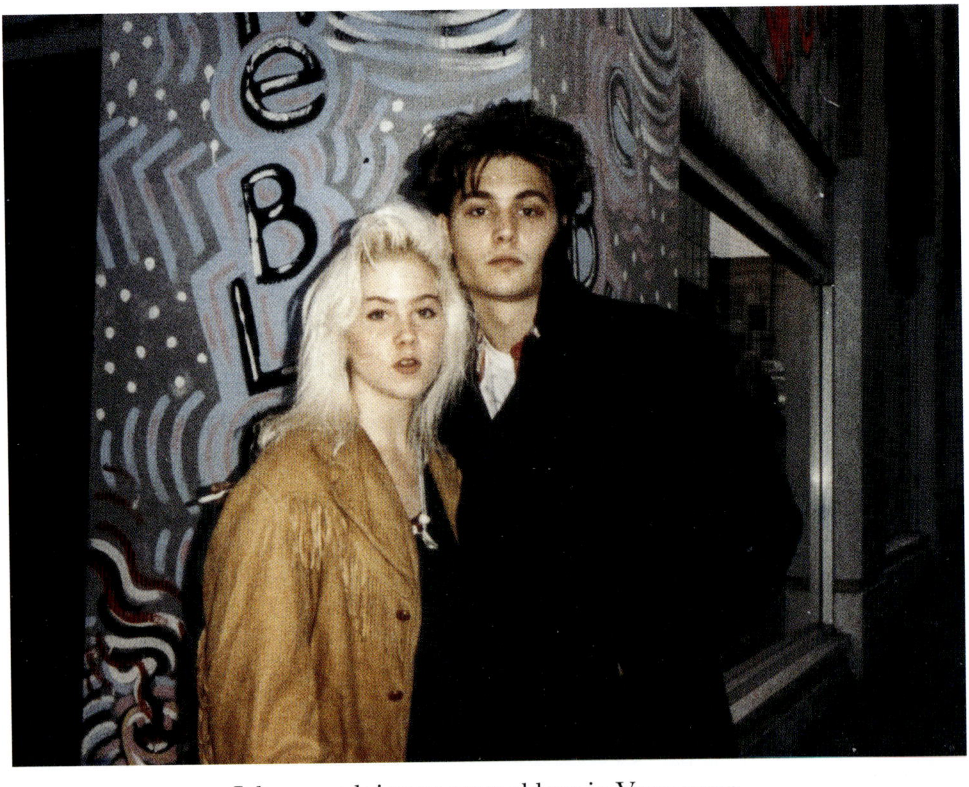

Johnny and sixteen-year-old me in Vancouver.

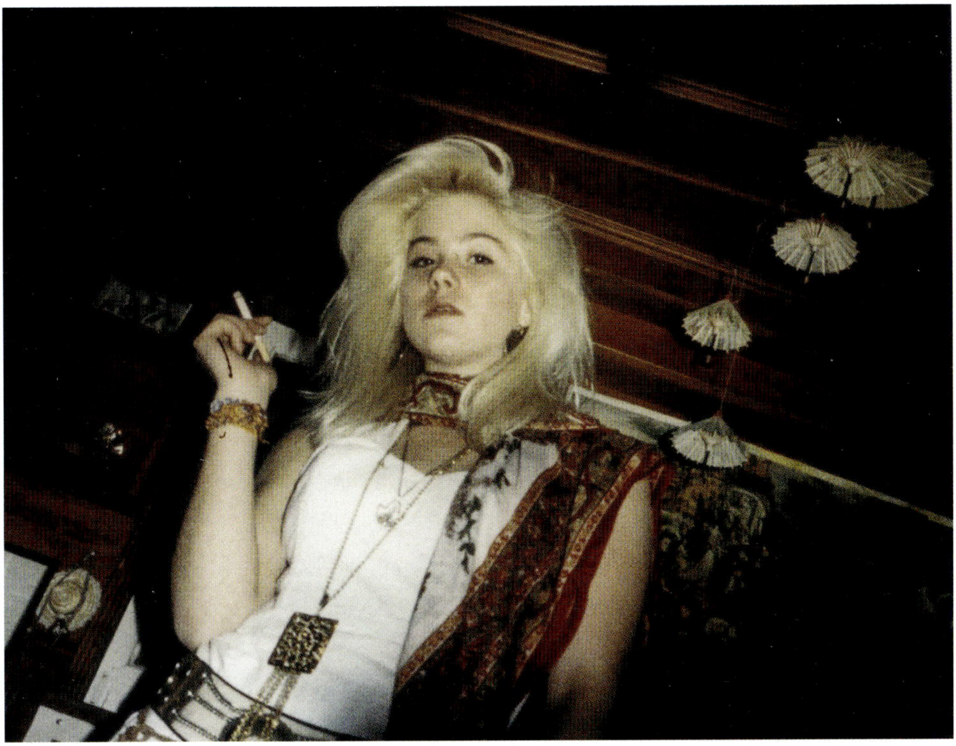

"Take one thing off." —Coco Chanel. Me in my Lookout Mountain bedroom.

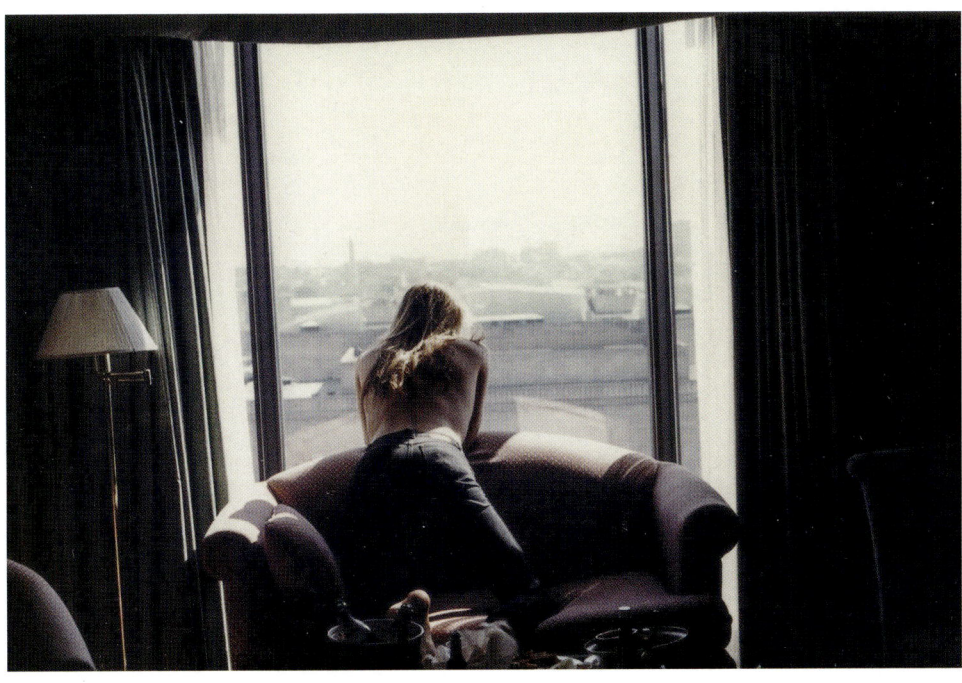

Me or my doppelganger, Sebastian Bach?

THURS NOV 2, 1989
2:20 PM PARIS.

GREY PAREE

In a place not knowing of my world,
I stare out at the dancing rain.
On a balcony I sit, six floors high, alone
Somewhere, out there, you sleep the day away,
maybe someway I'm in your dreams.
So on a balcony I sit, six floors high, alone.
Tonight you will sing for all but me,
But I am there, haunting but true
But on a balcony I sit six floors high, alone.
Ah, the rain has begun a thunderous flight
to salute those of us less fortunate ones
yes on a balcony I sit, six floors high, alone,
How I could soar if I leapt from here
No more pain, no more grief...... no more you
So on a balcony I wait six floors high, alone.
I know you feel me, for I feel you
It's like a plague we've been diagnosed
On a balcony I sit six floors high, alone.
It's getting quite cold on this thursday morn.
So I will go inside
and close my windows to the world,
and my balcony
and I will drown in my thoughts
within these walls of this generic room
and lay in my bed six floors high, alone.

Grey Paree poem.

Sunday Nov, 4, 1989
11:59 PM

2

Well I could lie and tell you Paris was phenom. But it wasn't. Marie went to see Bass. Mariah, like always, layed shit upon my happiness, and it rained every day. Life really makes me laugh. I don't think I have to explain why. I really do have to laugh it off though. Sadistic but true. Although I'm blessed, my life, as far as romance is concerned, hasn't proved itself as worthy of that title. Strange but true I received a call from Mosuier Wirth. Reading his undying emptiness without me in the vicinity. Actually he just said he missed me. Oh poor boy. He's just so "lonely." But me? oh shit, who knows how I feel. I feel comfortably numb. Bye for now,

A diary entry from my grey time in Paris.

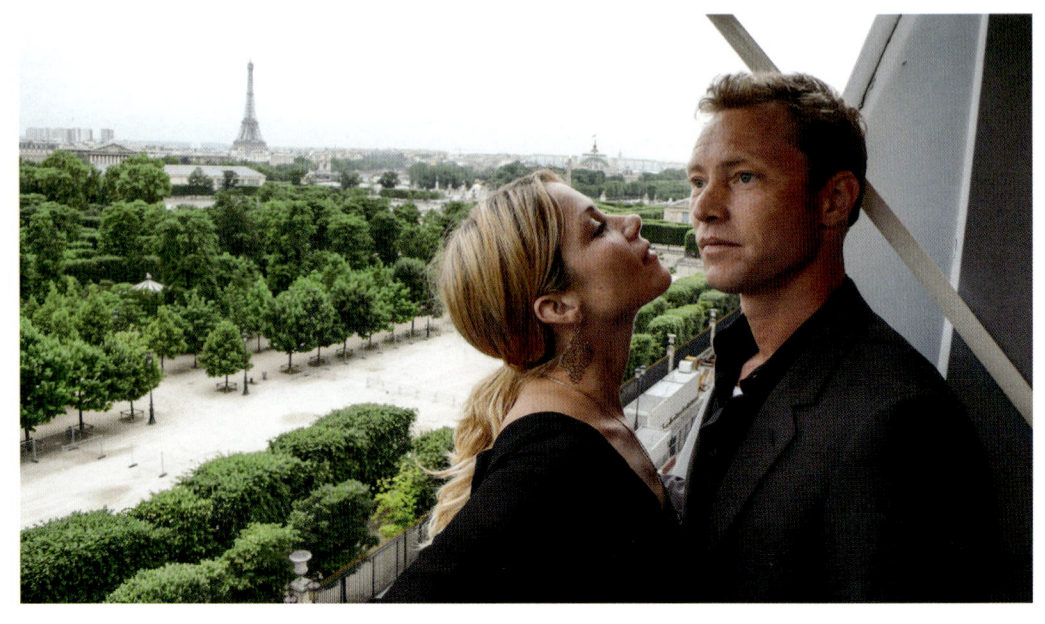

My kismet love.

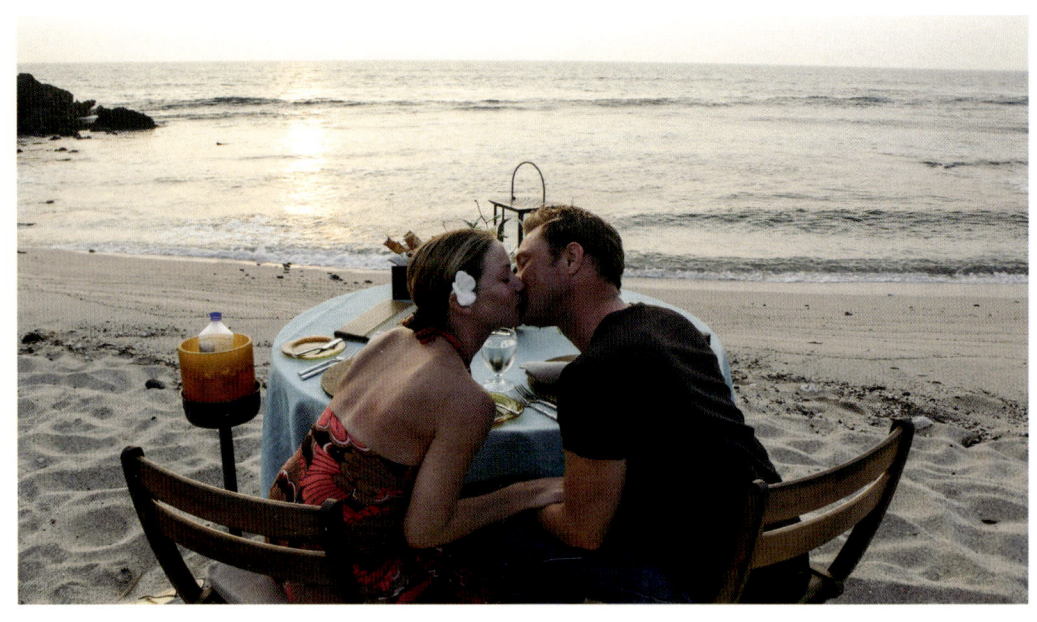

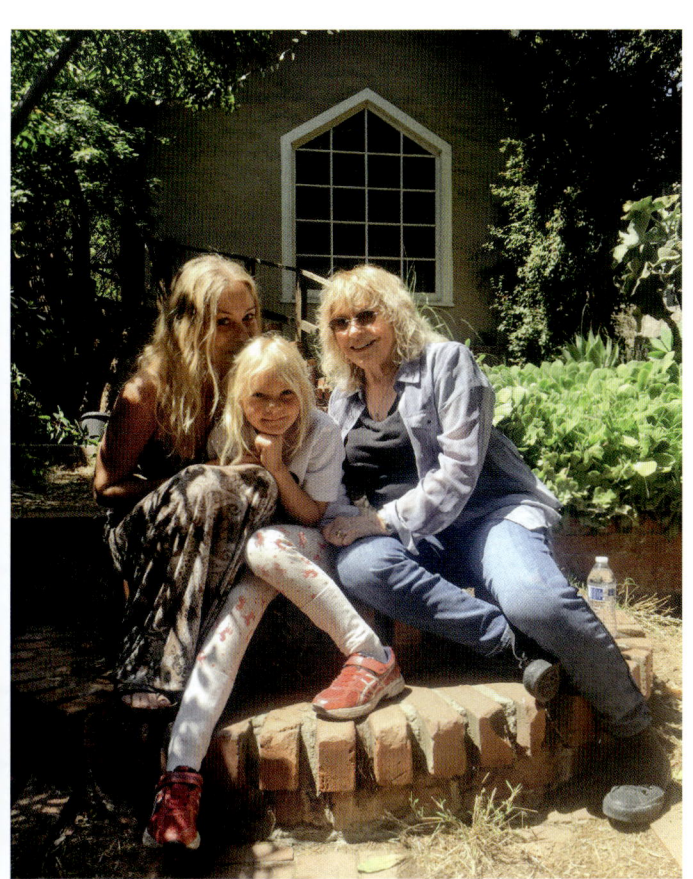

Three generations at the Lookout Mountain house!

The tiny door I had to walk through to get to my childhood bedroom. So glad Sadie got to see it.

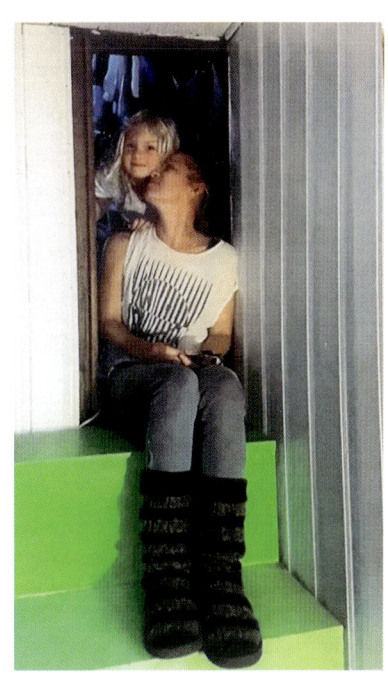

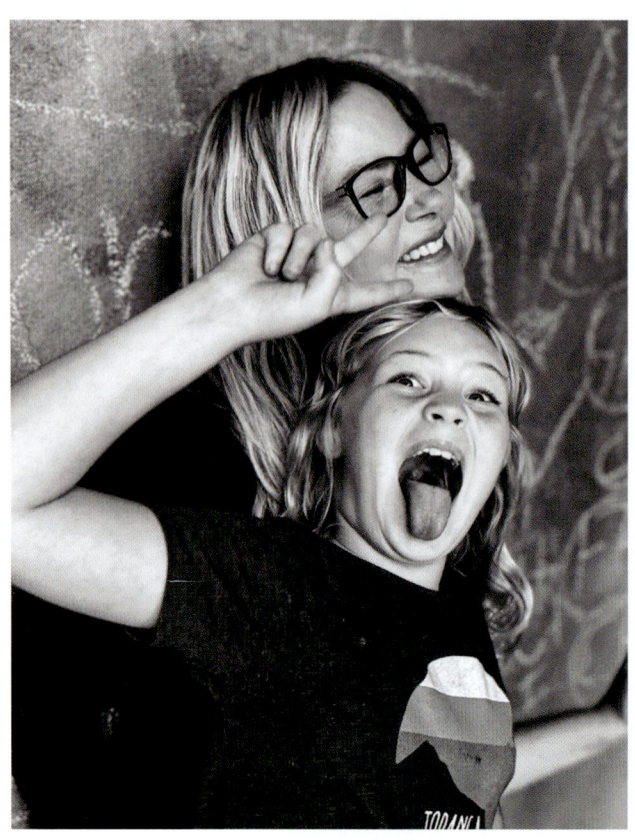

Emmy night at home in 2020. My first Emmys for *Dead to Me*.

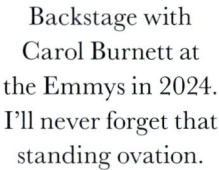

Backstage with Carol Burnett at the Emmys in 2024. I'll never forget that standing ovation.

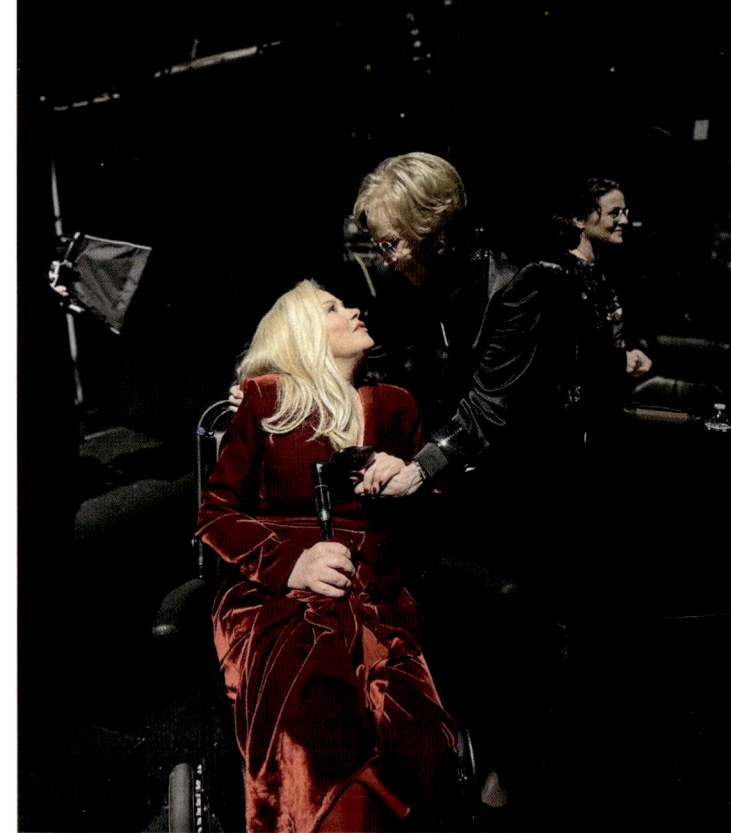

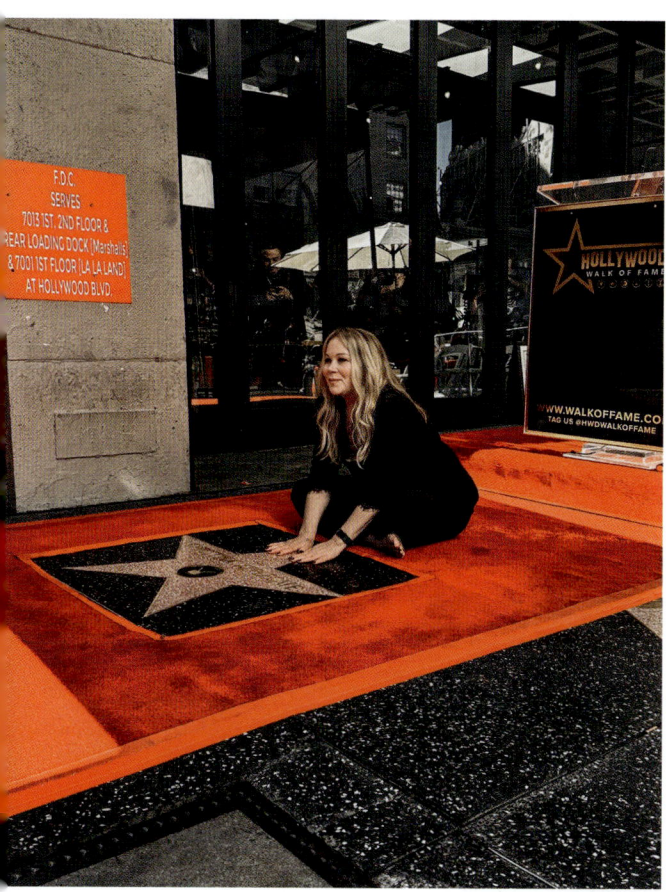

One of the coolest things that's ever happened to me.

Star, fucker, forever!

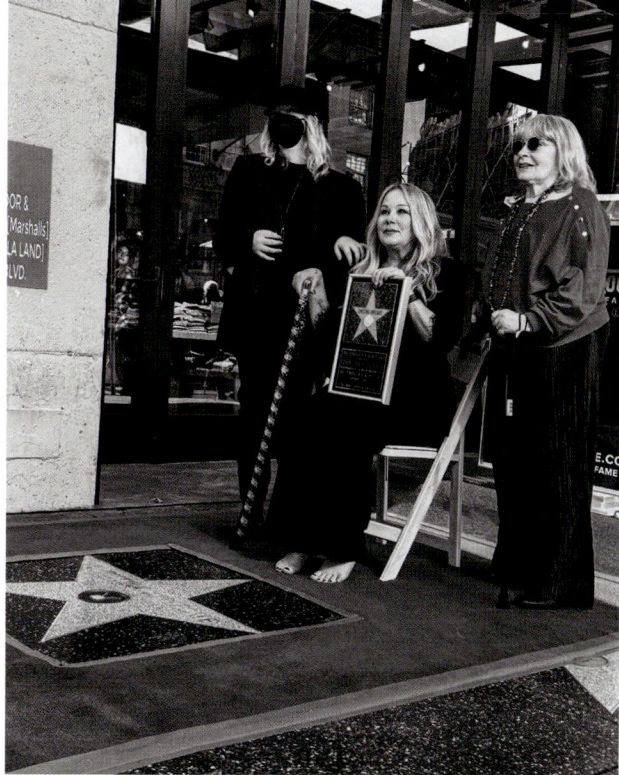

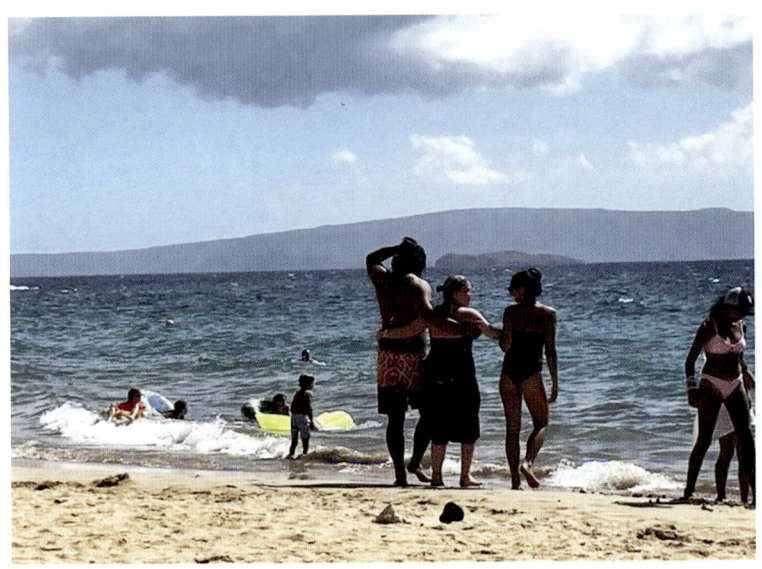
In Hawaii with friends. My first walk down a beach with MS.

night. As we drive, outside the winter's unrest rattles the car. It's bleak, and freezing, and I'm terrified, though part of me still thinks I can save this man, save myself, save the relationship and get the love I want, a love that is also, and quite perversely, something I feel I don't deserve.

And then, as we approach the motel, he leans over to me, his breath hot on my ear.

"If you don't come with me when we get to the motel...," he whispers, before saying something so evil I can't bear to repeat it. I know that he will hurt the people I love most if I don't go.

The air in the car curdles. I can taste the hatred in his mouth, the stale, peevish nastiness frosting the inside of the windows. I'm trapped; my mother hasn't heard what he's said. If I say it out loud, what will she do: call the cops again? We had our chance, and now I'm stuck here with him.

Part of me wants to calm him down, and part of me is still that little girl who's in love with him. The rest of me is pure terror.

There's no way out. We turn into the motel parking lot. I see that my hands are shaking again, almost imperceptibly, like the ripples of a distant earthquake.

The car stops. My mother waits. He gets out of the car. He looks back at me, and I know I have to go with him. Before he can shut the door, I get out of the car.

Now my mom starts screaming.

"What the fuck are you doing?" she shouts. "What's wrong with you?" All the years she couldn't save herself from Lala seem to come to the surface of her voice. She's screaming for me, and for herself.

"I'm just going to go in there for a little bit and sit there," I say, shaking.

"You go in there and I'm never fucking talking to you again," she says.

"I gotta go, I gotta go," I say.

I am looking at her, back into the low glow of the car, praying she can see the two words my eyes are trying to convey:

Help me.

Because I feel I am going to die tonight; everything in me feels that. But the power of my sad eyes fails me. She cannot understand what my eyes are trying to say. This is not a language any mother can, or should be able to, understand. Her daughter is walking away toward a fifty-buck-a-night motel with this man. What can she do? She has seen the future, and it can't be stopped; she has lived this in the past, and for many years couldn't stop that either. I am an adult now. I can make my own choices. This is the choice I've made, though perhaps just as she understood once, it's something that was no choice at all.

Incredibly, my mother starts up the car and drives away. My eyes couldn't reach hers. It is not her fault, just as it is not mine.

You with the Sad Eyes

* * *

The motel room is as disgusting as you might imagine: brown, mottled, unkempt carpet; a gross bedspread that has God knows what living in it; a TV that's mostly static; a single broken brown chair in the corner; a yellow rotary-dial telephone; orange, too-thin curtains; a Gideon's Bible in the side table... Actually, the room was so bad it was probably a *Jeff's* Bible.

I don't know why a joke about a Bible comes to mind now when I think about that horrible moment. Perhaps I'm still trying to save that girl with funny.

The man throws his shit down on the floor, takes a step toward me. My body hits the bed, hard. I'm paralyzed there. I know I'm doomed, that I probably won't live through this.

This is the end.

He sits down in the chair and looks at me. He smiles, a sick, evil smile.

"Another evening ruined by you," he says.

I can't move. My body feels like concrete, like a great lost weight falling to the bottom of a six-thousand-fathom ocean.

"Can I call and say I'm here...?"

I think of it this way: if I call my mom, perhaps the waver in my voice will communicate what my eyes couldn't convey — that I need help. They say a new mother can tell the cry of her child above all the others in a packed newborn nursery. Perhaps mine will hear my cry in the quaver of my voice, in the words I *don't* say, in how far I stray from what I would usually say to those words I *do* choose to share.

I have to tell her. I have to tell her to get me out of here...

"*No!*" he shouts.

Then he reconsiders and says words that still haunt me; they will always haunt me.

"Actually, you can call whoever the fuck you want," he says quietly, firmly, nastily. "It won't matter." I see in his eyes that I'll be dead before they even get here. "I really don't give a shit."

I watch him walk across the room and go into the bathroom. I hear him punch the mirror, hear the shattering glass. I watch as he brings out a shard. He comes toward me. I feel something cold on my neck.

My newfound sense of the possibility of survival falters. I realize with horror that he's not going to kill me yet, that in fact something worse is going to happen before he does so.

I am so terrified I realize I'm calm. Time moves imperceptibly, crawling along like a sloth. My blood stills. My mouth, dry from terror, loosens as though my mother has passed me my morning juice to wake it up. Is there an edge to me now, suddenly, the first flickering of a survivor?

You with the Sad Eyes

Something about his threats rings hollow, and the cold edge of the broken mirror sparks a surge of adrenaline, as though my kidnapper has brought me a warm meal after weeks of abandonment. No, I'm not going to die tonight. It's in my hands now.

I reach for the phone, but it's a mistake.

"I told you no. I told you if you went to the phone you'd be fucked," he says, holding my face to the bed while with the other hand he yanks the cord out of the wall. I can't breathe.

From behind my eyes, I feel a torrent, and suddenly I'm crying, hard, uncontrollably. I want to be strong, to kick back, but this man is stronger. Do I still hold out, deep in my reptilian brain, the hope of redemption for us, for everyone? This is the curse and the power of women: we can find forgiveness even in a place of irredeemable violence.

Then his tone changes again.

"You know what, I'm not going to kill you," he taunts. "Take off your clothes."

I think I'd rather die than have sex with this person right now.

He makes me get in bed, makes me get on top of him. I am crying so hard.

I think I'm going to throw up.

I'm lying on top of this monster that I'm supposed to love. And the weirdest thing is that the smell of him, a smell I have come to associate with home, overpowers me... and yet now its source has promised to kill me, and I fear he's going to rape me.

"Please, please, please," a voice is saying. "Let me go. Please let me go." It is my voice, a famous voice, one known to millions of TV viewers, but unrecognizable in its fear, and heard by no one save this man who I have told myself I love.

This isn't my time. Surely this isn't my time. Not today, not today, not today.

My prayer is answered, I don't know how. He relents a little and momentarily lets me go.

"Okay," he says quietly, "put your clothes on, call a cab, and get the fuck out of here."

When I look back, I realize something: he seemed to have gotten great enjoyment out of treating me like that. He seemed to take pleasure in making me truly believe he was going to kill me. My all-consuming fear appeared to satisfy him. I felt like he could see the terror in my face, how his anger made my body useless. It's as if making me cry, making me feel terror, and my showing him that terror in my eyes had been enough for him. It seemed as though he'd gained some power, as though that's what he liked.

Feeling the loosening of his grip, the wilting of the glass in his hand, the sense that something has run its course, I push myself off of him, throw on my clothes, bolt to the door, and run to the front desk.

The place is shut up for the night. I see no one.

How long do I have before he comes to get me once again? Surely he's not going to let me escape a third time today.

I pound on the locked door of the motel office. Nothing. The guy who runs the place, who I imagine also lives here, is probably in a back room, drinking his whiskey in his dirty tighty-whities. Who knows? He might be watching me on TV.

I'm banging on the door, shouting, "Help, help, help!"

Finally, I see a light. A door opens. The guy appears.

"What's all this noise?" he asks.

"Call me a cab," I shout. "Please call me a cab."

He seems confused.

"Hurry—before he comes to get me!" I'm screaming now. "Hurry—before he comes to kill me."

This new verb, "kill," does the trick. He bolts back into his quarters and then comes back. He opens the office and lets me sit by the door.

The cab takes forever. As I wait, I realize that my nails are digging into the vinyl chair. Eventually, the man says, "There's a cab coming." He seems to recognize me, but perhaps I'm imagining it.

The cab arrives. I throw myself into the back seat and hide down low.

It feels like years, but I eventually get back to my grandmother's house. Everyone is asleep when I arrive. I ring the doorbell over and over and over and over and over. Finally, my mother opens the door, and I fall, right there in the hallway.

I just fall.

I wish I could say it was the end, but as is too often the case, it was not. Despite what happened in that motel—not to mention that my mother and the rest of the family were horrified at what they'd seen—we stayed together. The fact that I couldn't flee gives me endless compassion for women who can't find a way to escape.

The day after, he called.

"I have no money and no food," he said. "And I need some way to get back to L.A." No apology. According to him, that night had been my fault. I had almost ruined his camera film by turning the light on. I was the one to blame, hence I had to pay for it. I had done this to him, and I owed him a flight and a hotel and everything else in between. His luggage had finally showed up, so I sent it over with some cash.

I got him out of there. At least then I knew my family would be safe.

Eventually, he took a bus to Chicago and somehow got back to L.A., back to my house.

* * *

You with the Sad Eyes

Saturday, December 26, 1992
I cannot feel the freedom
Let me touch him — love him
But the chain around my neck is
tight.
Tug tug at my soul
Make me love you.
But can't I love him
He who will not whip me
But feed me flowers
And bathe in wine
And rub my temples
But I get the beating
A lighter to my eye
Blood. Yet I cannot stop!!!

In the early nineties, I made a movie called *Across the Moon* in between call times for *Married...* In it I play the girlfriend of an incarcerated guy, played by Peter Berg. The film was shot in L.A., as well as in and around Palmdale on the edge of the Mojave Desert. By now, the relationship had me so broken that physically I was wasting away — during the month it took to make *Across the Moon,* I went from a size 4 to a size 0, maybe less. I kept it all from the world.

One day he came to the cabin with my friend Bill.

The fighting commenced yet again. We ended up in the basement arguing violently. Bill called his sister from upstairs, and she later said she could hear me screaming even though I was nowhere near the phone.

"Bill!" she said. "You gotta go help her."

"But he'll kill me," Bill said.

At one point, I ended up on the ground, and my head slammed into the floor. The fall left me with a skull that was so swollen that when I went to work, the hairstylist on *Married...* had to make my hair bigger so it wouldn't show when we were filming. I told the stylist what had happened but kept it from everyone else—professional, professional, professional.

I couldn't believe I'd been through all of this yet again. I hate even recounting it. I want to shake that twenty-two-year-old, wake her up. But that's too easy to say now—she was bound by a situation from which she couldn't escape.

I have to forgive her. I do forgive her.

I would wake up every morning with my stomach on fire from all the stress I was going through. On a break from shooting, I headed home to L.A. from the desert, only to find him stinking drunk. The next day as I was leaving to go back to set, we got into yet another terrible fight, so bad that I just lost control of my body entirely and fell halfway down the stairs on my way out to my car. Seeing the state I was in, he offered to drive me the two hours back to Palmdale. But on the freeway, he kept driving toward the center divider, like he was going to kill us.

I know now that he wanted to see the fear in my face; it seemed to placate him every time. But how much longer could this go on?

A few nights later he called to tell me that he'd met someone.

It felt like a tiny chink of light in the darkness. Now I didn't have to decide. Now I didn't need anyone to save me. Now I could finally escape.

He was to move out immediately, take his stuff and be gone.

At the time, a dear friend of mine, Gary, was dying of AIDS. I went to his house with a bunch of his other friends to say goodbye while my boyfriend was supposed to pack up his shit and leave.

We were all there, loving on Gary, drinking wine and celebrating him as he lay, his eyes open, but not there, not in any real way. I had bought Gary a crystal ball years before, and at one point, I put it next to him on the bed. And even though he was far gone, we all watched in amazement as he reached out his hand to the crystal ball. His fingers moved around it.

"Oh, honey," I whispered. "I love you, Gary. Goodbye."

When I got home that day, once again I could see it and taste it, that scent of malevolence, of something so far off normal that no words could save it. Far from having left, my boyfriend was lying asleep on a futon in the living room. Next to him was a bottle of tequila and a bottle of Vicodin, both seemingly left open, I realize now, for me to think he'd swallowed a whole bunch of pills.

But I was just so exhausted from being with Gary that I heard myself very quietly say, "Okay, all right, whatever." I poured myself a shot of tequila and lit up a cigarette.

I sat there, watching him sleep, hating the fact that he was still there. As I smoked, the phone rang, and when I answered, my mom's voice came through.

"Gary's gone."

I started to cry, and as I did, this creature rose up from the futon and looked at me with that familiar stare, the look that seemed to say, "You're dead."

Here we go, I thought. I was used to it now.

What happened next was like a dream. Something was off, as though he had indeed taken a bunch of pills and tequila. He picked up my car keys and started to walk toward the door. But he was stumbling around, walking at an angle.

"Don't take the car," I said. "You'll kill yourself." I was trying to physically stop him from leaving. "You can't drive right now. You can barely walk..."

But he was too strong for me, and he pushed past

me out to the car and drove away. I immediately called the cops, telling them what kind of car and the license plate.

"You have to stop him," I said. "He's going to kill someone."

They said there was nothing they could do.

I was desperate and called a friend of his in San Francisco to see if he'd contacted them to say he was on his way. As I was on the phone, he suddenly appeared in the doorway. He wasn't falling around anymore. He seemed sober now, focused, like he had a mission, like it had all been a ruse.

I was relieved, and not. A part of me wished he had gotten into a car accident and died. The truth is, in my mind, I planned his death every day—that's why I never had a gun. I used to think, *I'll put a bullet through his head if he doesn't put one through mine.*

I'm fucked, I thought. *I'm fucked.*

"How much did you have to drink tonight, Christina?" he said.

"Not that much..."

"You did too. You're a fucking alcoholic."

"No I'm not. Fuck you. My friend was dying. I'm not drunk. I drove..."

Before I could finish, a cigarette lighter flew across the room and split the skin above my eye wide open. I still have the scar. Blood was shooting out of my face, splattering all over a sleeping bag I'd grabbed.

"Oh, you want to be a little drunken *whore*?" he said, seething.

Now he was coming at me, the bottle of tequila in his hand. He grabbed me, pulled my head back by my hair, and, rather than beat me with the bottle, as I thought he might, pushed me to the floor, where he held my nose and poured the entire bottle of tequila down my throat.

The liquor burned. I felt the room sway. Was this really happening? I gagged on all the liquid in my stomach, hoping I could throw it up quickly, before I got severe alcohol poisoning.

But despite my almost instant and debilitating intoxication, I wasn't stupid; I knew how to work my shit.

"I'm sorry," I said. "I deserve it. I'm sorry. Deserve it. I'm sorry." I was sitting up now, placating him, playing him.

"I need to call my mom back, tell her everything's okay," I said. "She heard some of this, so..." I was insinuating that she might be on her way already.

He sat off to the side, his fervor yet again dissipating a little once his behavior seemed to have had the desired effect.

I called my mom, and I said to her, over and over, "Oh, no, I deserve it. I'm sorry you had to hear that. I deserve it, I deserve it..."

But it wasn't my mom I called — it was my security guy. As my fame had grown, it had become imperative

You with the Sad Eyes

that I have someone who would keep the crazies at bay, and I'd found a guy who once worked in an L.A.-based SWAT team. He was even part of the team that arrested O.J. Simpson.

He was a seriously badass motherfucker, and because I kept calling him "Mom," he knew.

That guy got into his car, put a light on top, and made it from Canyon Country, more than an hour away, to my log cabin on Lookout Mountain in less than twenty minutes.

When he arrived, he ran up the eighty steps as if in one bound. Coming through the back door, through the kitchen, and into the living room, he found my boyfriend sitting on the couch as though nothing had happened, and me mostly unconscious, in and out and incoherent. Each of my breaths was apparently separated by an eternity, he told me later. "Almost dead," he said. "You were almost dead."

I was fading, but when I was awake, I was whispering, "Pretend I'm sleeping. Pretend I'm sleeping."

My security guy didn't need any more information.

"You need to leave now," he said to him.

"Who the fuck are you to...?" he started to say, making as if to fight him.

Bad idea. It didn't take my security guy long to get him the fuck out.

* * *

For the next couple of months, SWAT guys sat outside my house twenty-four hours a day with all the artillery you could possibly imagine in their trunks. One of them, a guy named Bob, kept saying, "I keep seeing that asshole drive by. Can't I just shoot him? I have a license to actually kill a person."

I realized a license to kill a person was not a thing, but still, I found it comforting.

"Do whatever you want to do," I said.

I'm sorry if I keep leading you to believe this is the end of the story. You'd certainly think that it would be…alas.

After I kicked him out, the guy moved into a place in a really nasty part of L.A. It was so bad that he was sharing a room, sleeping on a bunk bed. I felt awful, yet again. I even brought him Christmas presents. I was still trying to be the best girlfriend. I showed up as a surprise at his apartment, dressed in a full Santa suit with the beard, the long white hair, fat tummy, boots. I was carrying a huge satchel of presents over my shoulder.

Because that's something he had never had: a real Christmas. He had ruined mine every fucking year before that, but still I couldn't fully see that, or really know it. I wanted to be looked at as an amazing friend who did all these great things.

And yes, I can hear the bargaining in my words. This is how the cycle works.

That man never took full responsibility for anything he ever did. I think I was partly brainwashed for years, somehow thinking that what happened between us was my fault. For years I thought, *As much as I sit here and ridicule him, and blame everything on him, there's this little part of me that added some fuel to the fire in those situations.* My mind would say, *You did, Christina, you did.* I have always had a strong sense that I need to take responsibility for everybody's pain, and I never want to place responsibility or fault on anybody else about anything.

It's fucked up—I know that. I can't bear thinking that I'm too bold or think too highly of myself. I will forever be that girl passing the 20th Century Fox lot and innocently saying, "Oh my god, that's so weird. That's where I live!," and there will always be that silence, and then my friend will always be saying, "You're doing it."

It can take more than coming face-to-face with death to get out of a traumatic relationship. It's not rare for a woman in my situation to stay even when she had the chance to leave. Society often judges women for staying in bad relationships, but it's not as easy as all that. I've lived it. It can feel impossible to break free of these kinds of relationships right up until the moment it's *not* impossible. But for the terrible, seemingly endless stretch during which we stay, or leave and then return, perceptions are warped, feelings subsumed, and fleeing can be harder than staying because remaining in a pain that one feels comfortable in can be easier than facing the disaster of a relationship that's over.

More than all that, I think I was still so terrified, in fear for my life.

But there's another truth: I was allured by the craziness in him. I guess I'll never know the full truth of who he was.

There's a certain chaos that casts a shadow over all the relationships I've had. Not that they were all like this guy; it's just that they were lost souls who I thought I could fix. Over and over, I've picked men who didn't treat me very well because I lacked the kind of self-worth that denies such men any kind of sway or power. All too often a small voice in me agreed with them that I wasn't worth the love I craved. I stayed longer than I should have, and damage begat damage begat damage, until now here I am, lesions pulsing on my brain like broken stoplights.

No one should shame a woman for staying in a terrible situation like the one I faced. Because when we're in it, we really don't know what to do. We're scared.

There should be no shame in staying—please: we are already too hard on ourselves—but there is no survival in it either.

You with the Sad Eyes

* * *

After the real end, through the years he would send me mixtapes of music, things he'd painted from memory, even champagne bottle corks from bottles we had drunk together. It felt like he was always trying to get at me, to remind me he was still around.

In early 1993, a young actor right out of college by the name of David Boreanaz made his first credited appearance on TV in *Married… with Children*. He played Kelly's love interest on an episode called "Movie Show." I met him first thing that workweek. David and I quickly became friends—he was funny and kind and we would pass our lunchtimes together. When, on Thursday of that week, yet again something happened with my boyfriend, I called David, even though I'd known him for only four days.

"I can't be alone in my house," I said, and David showed up at the log cabin to keep me company.

David made me feel safe in my house, and a few days later, he and I started a thing. We dated for a few months, and even though it didn't last, he helped me eventually leave. I adore David for that. Thinking back, I can't say enough how much I appreciated him for being the reason I was finally able to get back to normal.

After my time with David ended, I went from

relationship to relationship, as if being with someone was insurance against going back to that terrible boyfriend. With enough time apart, I felt his hold on me wane, until finally it was done. I haven't heard from him in decades.

With him finally gone from my life for good, I sold the log cabin. I couldn't deal with the memories of being there anymore. The place was filled with his ghost and what he did to me: the lighter thrown, the blood spilled, the tequila forced down my throat, the nights he'd disappear into his film studio, which he'd set up in our guesthouse, and stay there till five in the morning, leaving me alone and wondering who this man in my house really was.

Living there became too painful. The vibes were wrong; the slip-and-slide gang had mostly moved on, but the wisteria still bloomed and does to this day, its roots so strong, its blossoms so beautiful — a reminder and a symbol of my resilience. But the entire property also felt small and claustrophobic, and the eighty steps from the street felt like eight hundred some days.

So on the back of the success of *Married...with Children* and the movies I'd made, I bought myself a house farther up on Lookout Mountain, secluded and beautiful. It has a gate, and security, and a koi pond, and when you look out, all you can see are trees.

I still live in that house. With my daughter, and my

chimes, my fireplace, and my nag champa... and with these memories, swirling around my bed at night, ghostly and perverse, and I'm wondering where everyone is, wondering what I did wrong, what I did to deserve what happened to me.

I don't know if this experience gave me strength. I only know that in the subsequent years, I found a calmness and a serenity. Perhaps I would have gotten there eventually, regardless of whether this had happened to me. I don't know if I can say that there was a big lesson from all of it, except that it happened, and perhaps by sharing it, someone else might be able to escape more quickly than I did, or else perhaps they might be able to listen more closely to the voice that tells them when something is terribly wrong.

I certainly learned to listen to my heart, to my gut. And ever since I haven't been controlled by anything or anyone.

I'm way too important. My opinions matter.

I am stronger, resilient, like that wisteria. What I went through brought me knowledge, a knowledge born out of being angry and scared.

In the years after all this, I found my footing, but I had to be constantly vigilant about how it screwed me up when it came to relationships. I wasn't looking for just any man, not looking for a father figure. I was looking for an equal. Before, I would attract guys who

I could control, or who controlled me. I was forever trying to please, please these men who seemed so unsettled in themselves.

I also learned not to sell myself short. I learned to have some respect for myself. If men I dated didn't see that, then they were the ones who needed a new perspective, not me.

Finally, I could see.

I haven't seen that boyfriend since. It was as if a ghost, an Amityville horror, washed up at the door of my beautiful cabin, a house that's long since been demolished and replaced with a monstrosity, its new owners unaware, I imagine, that once not so long ago a bunch of dickheads partied their asses off in all the zestful stupidity of a long-gone youth.

EIGHT

HAWAII

I've lost count of how many times my mother said to me, "It's you and me against the world." That puts a lot of pressure on a child and has probably loaned me a certain level of codependency. But more importantly, it has helped me develop the right safeguards against manipulation in this challenging business. It's a toughness that I want to teach my daughter, but I want all young women, especially in show business, or any business, to always know that they need you more than you need them. My mom would say it to me when I'd go to auditions, and I still know it to be true: they need me more than I need them.

As *Married...with Children* came to its natural conclusion, I found myself desperate to leave Kelly Bundy behind. I couldn't wait to take off the mask and be myself. I wanted to show the world, and myself, what I was capable of.

For the last two years of *Married...* I was wearing a wig because I had cut my hair short and dyed it a mix of black, cherry, and purple. I showed up with my new hairdo at a Fox event right before we were about to start filming the penultimate season.

"What's happening here?" someone said, a look of shock and horror on their face.

"We're getting a wig," I said.

I'd had blond hair down to my butt for more or less a decade but now I didn't care. There wasn't much else they could say because it wasn't as if I could suddenly grow my hair ten inches.

They needed me more than I needed them. It was me against the world, kid.

I'm grateful for *Married...*, grateful for the time I spent there, grateful for the lessons I learned, grateful for the family I had in Ed and Katey and David, but if I didn't get that girl away from me, I didn't know what I would do.

I needed to be me. But that doesn't mean I made great decisions. Right after *Married...* ended, a script came across my desk for a little movie called *Legally Blonde*. I didn't even audition or read for it or meet with anyone. I was done with the ditzy-blonde thing.

And to think, I could have had Reese Witherspoon Money™.

You with the Sad Eyes

* * *

Instead, I needed to escape.

It all began with David Faustino, my brother on *Married...* He had taken a vacation to Hawaii and returned with stars in his eyes. The way he described it made it sound both magical and one million miles away, both things I desperately needed. The friends David had made there—guys with names like Lawrence and Joji and Shaney Boy—sometimes flew to L.A. to visit him, and he would introduce me to them. I instantly fell in love with them as he had. They had a kindness, and a sly wit about them, as though that magical outpost in the ocean freed their souls from the kinds of concerns we mainland-bound suckers never seem to escape.

Each time his friends returned to Hawaii, I would be desperate to see them again, to find a place where goodness and love prevailed. I didn't know what paradise was until I went there. Given everything I'd been through, I wanted a paradise, and I found it in Maui, a place that would become my home away from home. When *Married...* went on hiatus, or when I didn't have a movie to shoot or a talk show to do, I would immediately fly there.

My friends in Hawaii filled my soul in ways I could never have imagined. Those beautiful people opened up their community to me in a way no tourist usually gets to see. Eventually, I found a place of my own where I could stay for a month at a time, and whenever I wasn't working, that's where you would find me.

The group of friends I made mostly worked at the luau, and I'd often show up just to watch them perform. At one point during a show, a canoe glided across the water with a flame on it, and my friend Shalia came out of the water in a white dress, so sinuous and gorgeous. I was captivated. Once the show was over, we'd sneak away to a nearby pineapple field to drink Bud Light and watch the skies, filled as they so often were with the most shooting stars you've ever seen, sparkling past our peripheral visions.

In those magical moments, these beautiful, kind, funny people became my family. The fact that I was "Christina Applegate" didn't matter to anyone, and certainly not to me. It was on Maui that I got my nickname, or what I think of as my real name, those two syllables behind which my true soul resides.

I'd go by myself, or bring my mom or a best friend. I'd share the beauty and friends I'd found with them and let them see the islands in a way that they'd never otherwise get to see them. But mostly I went alone, unseen, unphotographed, healing, finding a peace that had eluded me so far in my life.

For a while I was hanging out with—you know what I mean (fucking)—a boy on Maui. He was half

You with the Sad Eyes

Filipino, half Hawaiian, and had a sense of humor unlike anyone I knew on the mainland, and I worked in comedy. Ours was an easy, pure relationship, the kind those islands, and my happiness and lack of complication while there, made possible.

Thursday, April 1, 1993

The clouds may tear upon my face
But the sun is in my soul
The boy's fingertips have healed the wound
For now.
Still I am stale
Still I scramble
Not seeing what is right or wrong
...he lurks about my universe
Stabbing when I close my eyes
And spitting when I speak.
His hands are cold around my throat.
I cannot breathe.

I once brought an L.A. boyfriend to the islands, but my Hawaiian "lovah" wasn't happy about it. One time, we all headed to a club on Front Street—a club that has since burned down, to the agony of my heart and the hearts of so many on Maui—and while we all partied and danced, I was amused to see a woman walk past my L.A. boyfriend and playfully pinch his butt.

I was laughing, and my girlfriend, a beautiful nineteen-year-old Samoan woman, asked me what I found funny.

"Oh, nothing," I said, pointing vaguely at the dance floor. "It's just that chick, over there. She just pinched my boyfriend's butt."

Big mistake on my part. Without a word, my friend strode over to where the pincher was standing and hauled off and punched her, right in the face. Next thing I knew, we were all in the parking lot and this whole damn kerfuffle was ablaze, dust rising, fists flying, hair pulling — the whole nine yards.

At one point, there was a break in the action, and my friend came over to me. I must have looked completely horrified.

"What's wrong?" she said, out of breath.

"Honey," I said, "small problem. That wasn't her. Wrong chick. You literally punched the wrong person."

After a comic pause during which we both realized the ridiculous stupidity of what had just happened — and thankfully no one got seriously hurt — we burst out in hysterical laughter and ran to my car as fast as we could to get the hell out of there.

We've talked about that story a lot in the intervening years. My friend is older now — I hate how time does that—and she doesn't love that story as much these days. She's matured and doesn't live in that world anymore.

And that boyfriend with the pinched ass? Didn't last, of course, but hey, to quote my mother, "I never met a junkie I didn't like."

As much as I wanted it not to, real life still had a way of asserting itself on Maui.

> *April 18, 1995, Maui*
> *It's funny that the only time I feel inspired to write is when I am here. The only time I can reflect... My mom has cancer. She was diagnosed about 5 months ago. It's only temporary, I know that. I have to. She is going through chemotherapy now and it has been so hard on her and me. But there is such a great lesson to be learned here about life. Just how important it is to be happy. It sure isn't easy to acquire. I know that. I'm so disillusioned as to what it really is, though. I think it might be the sense of now. As simple as that may seem. Now isn't so bad as long as you are truly in it. Life is a gift. It's unfortunate that we all take life so for granted.*

My mom had breast cancer back in 1980, but this time, fifteen years later, it was ovarian. I was pissed off that she had cancer a second time—your mother's not supposed to have cancer; she's not supposed to not be able to take care of you. I resented it, in a way. I couldn't take it. I hated every second of it. She faced two years of chemo and ten surgeries, one of which removed half of her intestines.

She lost all her hair and became so fragile, immunocompromised, and sick. It was scary as fuck. I couldn't bear to see her like that. It crushes me that my own child is going through this now, in her own way.

But my mom also saved a lot of women when she went through ovarian cancer, because initially the doctors couldn't find the cancer in her ovaries, even though it was genetically marked to be ovarian cancer. In recent years, researchers have discovered that ovarian cancer can start in the fallopian tubes, and I understand that my mom's case was one that spurred on the research. For many women, by the time cancer is found in the ovaries, it's too late. These days, women also have their fallopian tubes removed when they have a hysterectomy, eliminating the danger of cancer in the fallopian tubes remaining undetected.

My mom survived, but it was a dark time, for both of us. I found myself struggling with dangerous thoughts even on my island oasis.

And now the saddest. A beautiful girl named Jennifer Justice took her own life on Sunday.

Although I wasn't extremely close to her, I'm affected all the same. What really affects me is that I know how she felt. All too often the thought of suicide crosses my mind. Almost every day. I am so damn tired of this life sometimes, it's scary.

At least I had Hawaii. Despite these spells of intense darkness, I was a happier, different person there, more myself than anywhere else. I was nobody famous. I was nobody. I wasn't only the survivor of my childhood. I wasn't only the woman who faced down a terrible boyfriend and found her freedom. I wasn't Kelly Bundy. I didn't even have to be Christina Applegate.

April 4, 1996, 9:45 p.m.
Just arrived in Oahu. Sitting in back of a stranger's truck on my way to swim with the dolphins. All is well in my kingdom. All is well.

PS. I rode underneath this blanket of stars tonight... I'm sleeping in a tent next to the crashing waves. It's so dark out, heaven on earth, heaven on earth. Deep calls unto deep and deep answers deep.

March 19, 1995, Maui

Here I am in Maui—my home, my soul, myself. I leave tomorrow. So sad. It's beautiful out right now. Just a few clouds that blanket the sun. The water like jewels, glistening, inviting. Soon the sun will set off to the right of Lanai. As it kisses the horizon I will see God. I will feel as small but powerful as the Universe intends. Ineffable.

August 6, 1996

I swam with the dolphins yesterday for about five hours. It was amazing the way we communicated. I felt joyous open exposed radiant clear... Today I felt high. I was floating in a surreal fog of absolute. Submerged in the warmth of God and my own power.

I was a new person. Through my healing on those islands, a new person emerged. She surprised even me.

These days, very little of Front Street on Maui survives, gone in the terrible fires of 2023. Every time I think of it my heart hurts. Many of my friends lost their homes; many are still displaced. This is made especially poignant as in recent months my hometown of Los Angeles has suffered catastrophic fires of its own. We evacuated during the worst of the winter fires of 2025 from an abundance of caution, but so many friends lost their homes here, all their possessions, their histories. My grief for Maui has only deepened in the past months, having faced similar losses here at home and seeing firsthand what people in Hawaii had to go through.

And my heart hurts for that time I spent in Hawaii for other reasons, too. After the terrible years with that abusive guy, I yearned for sanctuary, a place I could escape to, a place to heal.

I'm lucky I found it, out there at the very ends of the Pacific Ocean, the shooting stars jangling at the very edge of my sad eyes, somewhere out of sight.

NINE

FILTHY McNASTY

I hated the limelight, and everywhere in West Hollywood was bathed in it.

Then came the Viper Room.

I'm here to tell you that the Viper Room was the coolest club that ever existed. It was an otherwise squat and forgettable building at 8852 Sunset, right by Larrabee Street, built in the early 1920s. Originally it was a nondescript grocery store, though it would go on to have multiple famous iterations across the decades: at one time it was a nightclub, and then a bar called the Melody Lounge, which was something of a wiseguy hangout. Eventually, it became a club owned by and named for a legendary Angelino known to everyone as Filthy McNasty. Filthy McNasty was from Berlin, and his real name was the much less fun Wilfried Bartsch—you can see why he was happier to go by a new name.

Filthy McNasty's set the tone for what was to come. Famous people — everyone from Evel Knievel to John Wayne — loved the place because photographers were not welcome. In a city where paparazzi are as plentiful as fire hydrants, folks just wanted somewhere safe to hang out, away from prying lenses, especially in the days when celebrities cherished their privacy. They also knew they had to maintain it, so that when they did finally emerge, their presence would be something to talk about and might put bums in theater seats and movie halls. Nowadays, every famous person has an Instagram account where they share their most intimate moments the second they happen, but in an earlier time, it was imperative to keep a mystery about oneself, hence the advantage a place like Filthy McNasty's had in turning away the fame vampires.

In the eighties, Filthy McNasty's morphed into the Central, a jazz club that attracted performances by a young Rickie Lee Jones, as well as her musician friend Chuck E. Weiss. Rickie would write about a conversation with the third member of that famous trio of musicians, Tom Waits, in her hit "Chuck E.'s in Love."

When Chuck E. eventually persuaded Johnny Depp and others to buy the Central and turn it into the Viper Room, the owners were quick to reestablish the emphasis on privacy. They created a kind of speakeasy, an exclusive, secret-handshake sort of hangout that felt personal and familial, an escape from the crazy scene that dogged us everywhere we went in nineties Los Angeles.

Johnny also made sure that Chuck E. could still play there. This was a big deal, because Chuck E. Weiss wasn't to everyone's taste—he sometimes thrummed a washboard and told long tales in between his blues songs, accompanied as he usually was by his band, the Goddamn Liars. But I loved Chuck E., and he played at my twenty-second birthday party.

I'd been at the Viper Room's opening night back when I was twenty-one, and by that twenty-second birthday, the Viper Room had become my home away from home.

It attracted all the coolest people, cats you just wanted to be around. And it wasn't just celebrities: it was all manner of weirdos—"us weirdos," as we put it. Everyone was treated the same on the inside, no special treatment for being famous or known. Everyone was a character in their own way, like these four guys called the Millionaires' Club, who were never seen in public unless they were dressed in three-piece suits. Shannon and Carolyn and Tommi ran the Viper Room back then—they were the bartenders and managers, but really, they were its beating heart. Sometimes when Shannon was overwhelmed, she would make me help her at the bar. Then there was Sean G, who ran the front desk. These were my people.

The Viper Room was a list place—you couldn't get

in unless you were on it — but not for me. For me it was a home. I was there almost every night. Everyone felt like family, even the bouncers, like Big Ed, who was six foot five and could crush you if he wanted to, but who is also the sweetest man alive. I felt safe because Johnny had a standing policy of no assholes in the Viper Room. He wanted to create a place he could relax and hang out, and I felt the same way — it was the club where I could go and have drinks with a bunch of fucked-up fuckers, who didn't care who I was, and I didn't care who they were, as long as they were interesting and unfazed by fame. Most nights there weren't even paparazzi outside.

Everything, both inside and outside the Viper Room, was painted black. The air was always thick with cigarette smoke because Johnny would never have a place that you couldn't smoke inside. He once said, "I wish I could graft another mouth on my cheek so I could smoke more." There was a bar and booths, and my favorite spot, a secret room with one long bench opposite a wall that consisted of a one-way mirror, so you could sit in there on the bench and watch the whole club. It was a quieter spot where you could go and be alone, where you could corral your thoughts and take a breather. You could barely even hear the music. Carolyn or Pharel or another friend and I would sit on the bench and chat.

Johnny instilled a cherished level of privacy for

anyone, not just celebrities—the first rule of *Fight Club*, et cetera. It was our safe haven, a private place, and that's how it will remain.

> *August 15, 1993*
> *Last night at the Viper Room was a real turning point for me. I was elated and was feeling extremely close to myself... I'm happy, I realize that, even though the guilt is major... I realize how much better my life is without [my abusive boyfriend]. How free I feel. It's wonderful. How much time I have to take care of the important things in my life. Even though I am exhausted today... my heart burns with so much love for my life. And so it is.*
>
> *...*
> *It's too bright and patient*
> *For us to wallow.*
> *So let us be grown*
> *Let us all blossom and sit*
> *Under the Apple tree.*

Sometime in 1995, I joined a show at the House of Blues called the Choreographer's Ball. All the choreographers in Los Angeles and beyond would put on a huge, beautiful dance production. It brought a real dance culture to Los Angeles, which at that time was not a thing. I remember performing to "Black Coffee" and a Prince song called "How Come U Don't Call Me Anymore?" It was a wonderful chance for me to express myself through dance, something I'd done all my life, but not always to an audience.

Through friends I ended up meeting Robin Antin, a dancer and choreographer. We hit it off—she even moved into my house for a while—and out of that friendship came the Pussycat Dolls. Robin had been toying with creating a mixture of Bob Fosse, *The Rocky Horror Picture Show,* and burlesque, with some fake striptease thrown in for good measure.

But mostly it was Fosse, Fosse, Fosse.

Initially there were no singers, and we didn't even have a name. We'd dance to anything from Eartha Kitt to the music from *Kiss Me, Kate* and *Sweet Charity*. I described it back then as "a cross between Ann-Margret and James Bond girls." We would head to the dance studio I'd built in my house and work out the choreography. The Pussycat Dolls weren't taking any clothes off, but we were giving the illusion that we were taking something off, layers upon layers leading to more layers. It was suggestive in all the right ways.

To me, dance wasn't sexual: it was a spiritual expression of pain and glory and all the things in between. It was church. And I certainly never thought of myself as sexy. In my early twenties, we'd all go to Flaming Colossus, a club on Bonnie Brae near MacArthur Park in a seedy corner of downtown Los Angeles. (My drink of choice those nights was Southern Comfort because that was Janis Joplin's drink and I was obsessed with her, and still am.) One night, some guy said to a friend of mine, "God, Christina is the *unsexiest* person I've ever met." Why my "friend" thought she should pass this on I'll never know, but once again, a random comment from somebody I should have been able to ignore played directly into my insecurities. I was on the cover of *People*'s 100 Most Beautiful once, and I remember coming across a comment that said I wasn't beautiful: I was just chosen because I'd had cancer. Those feelings ran deep into my relationships and into the bedroom.

Not one time have I looked in a mirror—even all done up—and thought, *Oh, I look good*. Not once, never, swear on my life, from the first day I could think until writing this sentence. Sure, I've seen okay pictures, but I've always put it down to the hairpiece or the lashes or the lighting or the airbrushing. It's never me.

Over the years I have scrawled multiple phrases in lipstick on my bathroom mirrors so I don't have to look at myself. I read the words instead. If I fail and catch a glimpse, I feel sick. I've lived my whole life onscreen, but if I ever catch the shows or movies on

TV, my familiar internal monologue of "Fat, ugly, old" pushes its way in.

But dance...dance takes me out of my head and into my body. It's about being me.

Eventually, my friend Shannon, the manager at the Viper Room, thought that the Pussycat Dolls would be a perfect fit for her Thursday speakeasy night. Thursdays at the Viper already had a fun Prohibition-era feel—DJ Dean R. Miller had been playing early-twentieth-century music every Thursday for months, and folks would dress in fedoras and suits—it was gangster, but in the original meaning of the word. Shannon told Johnny about the Dolls, and he invited us to audition for a Thursday-night spot.

While he smoked his smokes, we did our thing. I remember dancing to the Eartha Kitt track "My Discarded Men." The Dolls were very old-school Fosse, making people think that they were seeing something risqué, when they were really seeing only the magic of dance. We had rhythmic gymnasts in our group and ballet dancers on point. There was one girl named Sia who would do her entire performance on point while holding a cigarette, taking her leg up high above her shoulder.

"This is so fucking cool," Johnny said when we were

done. "This is why I opened this place. This is so Thursday." And that was it. He loved it. We were part of the Viper Room's Thursday-night entertainment for the next decade.

We quickly became a phenomenon. It got so big that we would feature guest stars like Gwen Stefani and Christina Aguilera. Back then we were still lip-synching for fun, dancing to 1940s songs. So many women wanted to be part of it. It was empowering. They wanted to do new things, unexpected things. They wanted to feel something that they had never felt before without it being blatant or for someone else. And then the next thing we knew, we were at the legendary Roxy nightclub, and we were selling out shows everywhere we went.

That's when Jimmy Iovine told Robin that the Pussycat Dolls should really be a singing group, not just a dance group. And Robin, the businesswoman that she is, took the idea and ran with it.

We'd gone from playing the Viper Room to the Roxy. If you can create a singing group that becomes number one on the charts, hell yeah, Robin, go for it. I'm proud of her. I really am.

But I was also disappointed. The dancing had subtly changed — suddenly, there was a lot of butt, if you get my drift. The line to see us would be around the corner. I remember saying to Robin during one Christmas performance, "There's a lot of booty-touching going on." Things were off, but empire's got to empire. Robin arrived places in a Bentley now. Good for her, but it wasn't what I'd originally been a part of.

But hey, man, we got "Don't Cha" ("Don't cha wish your girlfriend was hot like me"). This was never a sentiment I thought of for myself, but Nicole Scherzinger and a few OG Dolls dominated. How cool is that?

By my mid-twenties, things were changing everywhere I looked. Being free and single and doing your thing was one thing but going to a club most nights was something that didn't entirely appeal anymore. Many of us left and never went back.

My life was altogether way too complicated by my mid-twenties for me to even think much about the Viper Room. I was all over the place, veering from dating to tending to my mother's health to God, of all things!

> *February 15, 1996*
> *Wow, it's been a long time since I took the time to reflect. Since the last entry I've been through a lot. Men, shit, etc. I'll start with the name list. Derek, Richard, Ryan, Dennis, Reo, Ashley... Once again I might have*

gotten myself into a bit of a drama. Not too bad, though. Oh yeah, Troy NYC New Year's. There might be one more. Although I can't really remember.

. . .

Mom went through a lot with the cancer but she's okay now. I found God and it's the best thing to ever happen to me. AGAPE! My life, my breath.

I take too many classes, do too many things. I think I'm happy. I don't really know anymore. My house is beautiful. Can't think.

As the 1990s continued, my diaries chart my growing relationship with spirituality and God. I discovered the Agape International Spiritual Center, which had been founded in 1986 by Dr. Michael B. Beckwith, a charismatic and brilliant man. The center is not traditionally "Christian" in that it draws from multiple sources, multiple faiths, and often from the more esoteric, Gnostic traditions, all in the service of "[teaching] how an individual may cultivate their own unique relationship with this ineffable Presence and live in conscious connection with It."

Agape resonated with me because my mom had

always raised me to believe in an interconnectedness, an idea that God and I, and I and God, are one.

> *June 13, 1996*
> *I trust in God. I surrender—I am one in the spirit around me. It's okay, God, I get it. I heed my own words. Know you are there. Amen.*

This surrender I was feeling pushed me into a fresh perspective on my life, one I'd struggled to find in the past. For me to tell my diary that I loved myself, as I did in June 1996, was such a different song from the one I'd been singing for most of my life.

But sometimes the gains I had made could ebb within a day. Such was the trauma I carried with me, and such is the struggle the faithful have when God seems absent.

> *June 18, 1996*
> *I know you are present, I know you are present, but I feel so sad confused and tired today. I have faith in you and in me. Help me let it all go. You don't have to move the mountains, you just have to give me the strength to climb. You don't have to move the stumbling blocks, but lead me on, God! Pull*

me through. I know I must embody the truth about you and myself but why do I feel so shitty? Is it because I lost faith today? Is it because I became fearful? I don't want to fuck this up—I AM THE I AM I AM GOD I AM DIVINE I AM LOVE I AM RADIANCE I AM SUCCESS I AM WHAT YOU ARE. Amen.

Back and forth I went, feeling filled with faith, and then feeling lost to doubt. Yet the underlying sense from those years was that faith had stripped away the worst excesses of my self-hatred and had begun to give me a glimmer of self-esteem.

TEN

RED WEDDING

IN THE EARLY SUMMER of 2001, I shot a movie with Cameron Diaz called *The Sweetest Thing*. Cameron and I clicked from the moment we met at auditions. I loved every day of working with her. It never even felt like work, and that movie was such an important source of joy in my life at the time.

During the movie, we take a road trip, and it was during these car scenes that we really bonded. When filming a car scene, the vehicle you're in is attached to what's called an insert car—essentially a truck filled with cameras and sound guys that's towing your vehicle on a process trailer to give the illusion that you're driving. Everyone in the insert car can hear everything the actors say, even in between takes, because there's no efficient way to cut the sound off while cameras are reset and positions retaken.

Cameron and I had learned all the words to a song called "Tales of Taboo," which we referred to as "Belgian Waffles" because of a particularly foul lyric. The song was by a performance artist named Karen Finley. We were filming up in Sausalito along a road that's used a lot for movies set in San Francisco, and we'd have to go all the way down the road, turn around, and come back. The whole process took forever, so in between takes our favorite thing to do was play "Tales of Taboo" on the car stereo and sing along to it as loudly as possible, causing the crew to cringe half to death because it's the dirtiest song you've ever heard in your life. I urge all readers to listen to it immediately and do as Cameron and I did: learn every word, and sing it at high volume whenever possible.

The wonderful Parker Posey was also in that movie, and when she heard us singing "Tales of Taboo," she offered a song of her own: "Fuck the Pain Away" by Peaches.

"Sorry, Parker," I said, "but compared to 'Belgian Waffles,' 'Fuck the Pain Away' sounds like something from *Blue's Clues*."

Again, there was this split personality between me on set and me at home. At work, I was having fun, screaming lyrics like "Make me a tit sandwich" with my new friend, playing one of two carefree party girls. At home, I was playing the role of a perfect bride-to-be, eating obsessively clean and not drinking, planning the "perfect" wedding for the "perfect" polished life. No tit sandwich for me.

Who wants to go to a wedding where no one is allowed to drink alcohol? I can't imagine there's a single person in the world who would choose to watch two people get hitched while stone-cold sober. But in October 2001, if you attended my (first) wedding, I was determined that you were going to be crystal clear mentally and physically for my vows.

It had to be perfect because he was everything my family wanted for me. My future husband had more than $3.50 in his bank account and didn't rely on me monetarily. Handsome fella. He liked sports, so Dad was on board. It felt like the right next step after years of disappointment. He disappointed no one, except maybe me.

If I went to a wedding now and they didn't serve alcohol, I'd leave, thank you very much. I don't mind if you're no good at drinking and want to abstain while you make your vows, but it's also not my fault you are bad at it. I had become such a health freak, and I was dead set on everyone being spiritual and clear, so I banned drinking before the ceremony.

I'm sure all my friends hated me. Or they had hip flasks hidden in their pockets. I hope they did. I think my poor bridesmaids snuck a drink or two when they were getting ready.

I picked a pretty house with a pool in Palm Springs as the venue outside the city. Jeffrey Best, the eminent event planner, helped create an experience that began well before the day. I made beautiful invitations, and when people accepted, they received a slim, leather-bound journal with a string wrapped around it that had all the available accommodations, the schedule of events, everything that you would need...and a notice that the wedding would be dry, of course.

Leading up to the big event I had been running every day, dancing every day. I'd quit drinking, was barely smoking cigarettes, nothing. (I would end up smoking a lot on the actual day.)

For the guests, I rented a truly beautiful hotel called the Korakia, a Tangier-inspired resort built originally in the 1920s by some random Scottish painter who wanted to be reminded of his time in Morocco, hence the archways, courtyard, fountain, and whitewashed walls. There were firepits and pools, every room was different, and oh: there were no TVs.

Also, no curtains. My soon-to-be father-in-law sought me out one morning and said, "Christina, I really need curtains..."

When he walked away, I felt my entire body

starting to convulse. I was a stressed-out, sober, cigaretteless bride.

"Tell everyone to go fuck themselves," I said to my assistant at the time. "I can't get him *curtains*. I am the *bride*. Have him go talk to someone else about his fucking curtains."

Suffice to say, I was a bit overwhelmed. All the man wanted was a dark room where he could get some rest.

At the rehearsal dinner, we served vegan Mediterranean food, and we all sat on pillows on the floor. All the waiters were wearing sarongs. To repeat, the food was vegan—so basically there was just a lot of hummus. Thankfully, the rehearsal dinner was not a dry event like the actual day, though drinking on a stomach of hummus doesn't seem amazing either. (Farts.)

I kept thinking, *This is* my *wedding. This is not your wedding. This is my wedding, my* perfect *wedding. This is what I would want a wedding to be like.*

I'd hate all that now. These days, I would insist on a TV, and a drink, and *fuck* sitting on the floor. I can barely get off my bed.

The actual ceremony was choreographed within an inch of its life.

The bride was not late. In fact, she was ten minutes *early*. Yes, folks, I was the bride who was ten fucking minutes early. I was also the bride who was pissed off at everybody else for being late. I was standing there with Dr. Michael Beckwith and a Catholic priest, who were co-officiating. As people showed up late, I hissed, "You've got to be fucking kidding me. I'm *ready*!"

No bride ever has said "I'm ready" in sober frustration.

We had written our own vows — mine were comical and lighthearted, whereas his were mushy-gushy, lovey-dovey, and no one ever accused me of liking that. I smiled gamely.

We had organized the whole thing using fake names, thereby avoiding the paparazzi, but still two people attended whom we didn't know. They were all dressed up and they even signed the guest book. Later, when I looked through it, I found a Polaroid picture they'd taken of themselves.

"Who the fuck are these two?" I said.

After the ceremony, I threw a huge cocktail reception. The dinner was created by Neal Fraser, a very talented chef who's worked with Wolfgang Puck and Thomas Keller, and who just so happened to have attended the Wonderland school with me. He served healthy miso soup and a blackened cod with a miso glaze and a seaweed salad. I thought it was delicious.

You with the Sad Eyes

I'm so sorry, everyone.

(Never fear—I'd added directions to the nearest McDonald's at the bottom of the menu. I'm not a savage.)

Once dinner was over, a fantastic and hilarious disco cover band called the Boogie Knights played, replete with fake Afros and real bell-bottoms. At one point, Stephen Stills got up and performed, but he played a little bit too long. I could sense that after the floor-hummus-rehearsal-dinner-no-drinking/TVs/curtains-miso-soup-seaweed-salad of it all, everyone just wanted to dance, so I hopped up onto the stage.

"You want me off, don't you?" one-third of Crosby, Stills, and Nash said.

I didn't need to say anything. But yes, I threw Stephen Stills offstage at my wedding. Don't hate me—people had been really digging him, and he'd been on fire playing, but I had a band ready to go, and I couldn't keep them waiting forever. You can't really dance to Stephen.

When people did finally leave, our parting gift to them was a double CD of every single song we'd played during the entire night. I had sat for days with my assistant going through what I wanted to play, from the second the guests walked in to the second they left.

I can't believe myself.

One of the reasons I'd insisted on a dry pre-ceremony is because I knew my friends all too well. I knew exactly what was going to happen. I just didn't want it to happen before my ceremony. Sure enough, on my wedding night, a bunch of people let loose, doing mushrooms and weird drugs and sleeping with other people's spouses. At six o'clock the morning after, I was lying in my marital bed, listening to the couple in the next room fighting because there was a woman in their bathtub with whom they'd had an intoxicated threesome.

The whole wedding was a master class in anal perfectionism. But that wasn't the worst thing. The worst thing was the moment I walked around the corner and into the ceremony. One of my favorite songs was playing, and when I looked hard at the face of my husband-to-be, I thought, *Oh fuck. Fuck, oh fuck.*

I have advice for women. If you go on a first date with a guy and you don't like his shoes, run — shoes are a telltale sign of whether or not a relationship will last. For our first date, he had shown up in boots, but not even cowboy boots. I think they were supposed to look like a cowboy boot, but they missed the mark by a wide margin. No one should wear such things, but especially not if you live in Los Angeles, California. The whole time, during that dinner, I remember thinking, *Those shoes are so bad. Bad shoes, bad shoes, bad shoes, bad shoes.*

But another voice said, *You're doing it again. This is the right person for you. He's got his shit together. He's attractive. He has a career.* We were just very different. I'm scrappy. I tell fucked-up jokes. I can be offensive and rough around the edges. He was none of those things.

I never considered stopping the wedding—for a start, I was halfway down the aisle. I kept thinking, *Don't be that guy. Don't be that guy. Don't be that guy. You're sabotaging. You're sabotaging. You're sabotaging.*

Because there I was in my custom gown, the center of this beautiful fucking wedding filled with all the perfect that you could possibly imagine.

And I knew right then that this man was not it for me.

About a year after I first met him, and a couple of years before we married, we'd gone on a trip up the coast to the Ventana hotel in Big Sur. We were together in a place where I was happy, but I also found myself alone a lot, as he often attended classes at nearby

Esalen Institute, just like Don Draper at the end of *Mad Men*. I stayed back by myself at the Ventana, on my hammock, writing in a new journal, with blank pages I'd hoped to fill with our happiness together.

> *August 19, 1998, 11 a.m., Big Sur*
> *It's wonderful to begin a new book. The other was so weighted down with pain and confusion. I needed to let it go. 5 years; I wrote there [in that previous journal] 5 years. No need to look back again. I understand it all. It molded me to who I am now in this moment, and I am grateful for that. So the unknown seems bright, exciting. I feel strong, I feel pretty good... How exciting. I can't wait to see how it will unfold. God is good, life is a gift. And so it is. Amen.*

I was looking out on the Pacific Ocean, swinging in a hammock, under perfect skies, and I was overcome with a feeling that I'd never had before. Not quite twenty-seven years old, and this was the first time I could actually think, *This is what happiness feels like?*

I'm staggered still that it took me nearly three decades to experience a moment of actual freedom, bliss, happiness. I know that the tyranny of "happiness," and the search for it, has warped our culture and made so many of us unhappy. Even so, to have spent all those years alienated from such a basic human need fills me now with sadness, a kind of root regret that is very hard to shake. Superficially, I was a success, but as the Pacific breeze gently moved that hammock, this elusive "happiness" appeared on the air for one of the first times in my life.

I wish I could have stayed in that place forever.

> *August 24, 1998*
>
> *Why do [we] have so many issues? I was so pissed. But all the truth finally came out... It still hurts. I still don't trust him altogether. What in me can trust? Why is it so fucking hard? He pulled something so shitty yesterday. It freaked me out. But he was rigid. I was looking for an out. A way out. A way out so I could feel free again, so I don't have to fucking worry about getting hurt again. I do want it to work. He certainly is a prize. But because he is so handsome it scares me. I feel sometimes that I don't think he's sincere. That he's full of shit. That he really doesn't feel for me the way he says he does. But what is that? Is it me not thinking I'm enough or is it truly a lack of sincerity? I guess I'll know for sure when he makes the real commitment.*

There I was, designer gown, sober, filled with hummus and sorrow, realizing I was making a mistake, and by 2006 we were divorced, and happiness eluded me once more, that fleeting butterfly, the hint at the edge of my vision that, once I turned my sad eyes to see, vanished.

ELEVEN

BING BANG BOOM

Before I made *ANCHORMAN*, I hadn't done much improv comedy—I always thought comedy was better when it was scripted, choreographed, "serious." My agents sent me the script, and I rolled my eyes. Too campy, too ridiculous; I wanted to be taken seriously. As I've said, I was a bit of an asshole.

I knew Will Ferrell was on *SNL* at the time, but other than that I had no real idea who anyone was, including the director, Adam McKay. I went to the audition begrudgingly, because my agents said it was a good idea. All I wanted was to have fun in auditions. It's not life and death—nothing is life and death in show business. Maybe my less-than-serious approach to that audition helped, because I did well, and I was asked back for a screen test.

So there I was, sitting in a room with three other

girls who had also been called back, each of us getting our hair done and prepping to go in. And then it was my turn. At one point we were running the scene in which Veronica and Ron are firing insults back and forth from behind the news desk while the credits roll. I liked sparring with Will; I had a great time with it. Then just as quickly we were done: bing bang boom.

"Okay," Adam said when we finished, "now do a take for fun."

My mind went blank. A voice in my head was saying, "But it's fun saying *your* words! I like saying your words!" By then, I was all too aware that I was in the presence of improv masters—Will Ferrell, who does it perfectly, seemingly without even thinking, not to mention Adam, who basically invented a whole type of improv, being one of the geniuses who created Chicago's Upright Citizens Brigade, where Amy Poehler, Horatio Sanz, and many other great comics plied their early trade.

But I had never done improv comedy. I'd grown up on a set where you say the words correctly, or you fail. You can't change even the smallest of things. We had to nail the script every single time.

"Just say whatever you want," McKay said, looking at me, waiting.

"Well," I started, with Will next to me. "Last night when we were together...I thought it was just your finger, but actually, it was your dick." That line came out of somewhere, I guess—my unconscious mind?

I'd slept with a guy once, and when I'd said, "You can put it in," he'd said, "I *am* in." That's how small his dick was. Art imitates life, I suppose.

Will and Adam lost their shit. Will broke, unable to stay in character. They wanted me for the job.

That wasn't the end of it, though.

When it came to agreeing on a fee, the studio lowballed me. I'm talking a stupidly lame amount of money. I said no.

"That's not going to happen," I said, and hung up the phone. They could go fuck themselves.

At the time, I was renting a beach house in Malibu, on Broad Beach, trying to get away from it all for a bit. My marriage wasn't going as planned. Apparently, a dry wedding with hummus was not the perfect send-off for a lifetime of happiness. I needed a win.

I got another call. This time it was Will and Adam.

"We want you. We want you so badly that we are going to take some of our salaries to pay you." For those two guys to make that offer meant so much to me. Women are almost never paid as much as the men they star alongside, but here were two titans of comedy offering me some of their share. I gratefully accepted.

I was touched, but I still thought this bizarre and over the top movie wasn't entirely my jam. Then I arrived to set, and found Steve Carell, Paul Rudd, David Koechner, Fred Willard, and Will and Adam. I was working with the best actors I've ever worked with in my entire career—except for James Marsden, but we'll get to that.

It was total dream stuff; I was in heaven.

Adam was no different on set than he was in the audition. He would often say, "Okay, now just do one take for fun." I still found myself thinking, *But it's fun saying your words. I like saying your words!* I tried to watch the others, to see what I could glean from how they did improv. Steve had *taught* improv, for fuck's sake, at the legendary Second City.

Then there was Fred. I thought Fred Willard was the funniest man on the entire planet. There's a scene in which Fred, playing Ed Harken, is in his office, talking to someone on the phone—we, the audience, don't know who—and Chris Parnell and I come swerving in with a pressing thing to tell him. Fred holds me off with a hand gesture, and I stand at his desk and watch as he talks into the phone.

"I have no idea where he would have gotten hold of German pornography. But you and I are mature adults—we've both seen our share of pornographic materials... Oh, you never have? Of course you haven't; how stupid of me. Neither have I—I was just speaking in generalities. Right, I'll stop by the school later, Sister Margaret..."

This was not in the script, and it was *exactly* my type of humor. Chris and I had to stand there and try not to crack. I barely made it through.

There I was with these masters of improv: Will, Steve, Adam, Paul, David, and Fred—that's just how their brains worked. Everything came from the central tenet of improvisational comedy, which states that whatever is said is accepted and built upon, the shorthand for which is "Yes, and..." For me, all this was new. On set I'd find myself saying to anyone who'd listen, "Teach me, Obi-Wan," but Steve Carell, especially, would just insist that I didn't need to be taught, that I could do it all by myself, which was such a beautiful act of belief in me. No one sat me down and held my hand and looked lovingly into my eyes and told me their wisdom. They just said, "Fuck you: you know how to do this."

So I studied what they did and tried to soak in their brilliance, until after days and days on set, my brain suddenly opened a portal and stuff just flew out. I had no idea where these thoughts were coming from. I was wholly unacquainted with the words that were coming out of my mouth. Truly, a part of my mind had unsealed and had grown a new and entirely surprising ability to improvise.

Sometimes when you're hired for a comedy movie and the man's the star, he's supposed to be the funny one, and you're not supposed to take away from that. This was not the case with *Anchorman*—I was able to go toe to toe with them. It was a master class I've taken with me on all my subsequent professional journeys.

Years later, I'd shoot *Vacation* with Ed Helms. I think it's one of the funniest movies I've ever done, but still I felt my part was written light. The directors listened to me and punched up the character of Debbie Griswold, Ed's character's wife, and I felt like an equal partner to Ed because I got to do my thing. Too often on set, you have to fight for your place with men because they don't like it when you're too funny. Another time I auditioned for a movie and I know that I didn't land the part because I was funnier than the lead actor. At the audition, I was getting bigger laughs than he was and the directors were cracking up at me, not at him. He was not laughing.

Then there's the flagrant mansplaining of it all. I auditioned for the role of Geneva in a Ron Howard movie, *The Dilemma*. The movie was to star Vince Vaughn, who I'd already worked with on *Anchorman*. At the audition, Ron suggested, "Why don't you guys just improv for a couple seconds right before you get into it?" Given our previous experience together, I was surprised when Vince looked me straight in the face and said, "Do you understand what that means? It means we're going to make up lines before we get into the scene."

Come on, bro, are you kidding me right now? I thought.

Needless to say, I didn't get the gig. Winona Ryder did, and I'm betting she improv'd the shit out of that scene.

You with the Sad Eyes

* * *

Improv can be scary, but bears are worse.

On *Anchorman*, during the bear pit scene, one of the animals we were working with was busy being a bear and I thought it moved in my direction. I shrieked, a totally reasonable response to being near a very large animal, however innocent it was. Someone—thank you, my savior—picked me up off my feet and swept me right out of there pronto. I was understandably rattled, my body shaking. May I remind you, those animals are not small! As an apology for my near-death experience—it wasn't near-death, but I'm a Drama Queen from Laurel Canyon™—the producers bought me a then state-of-the-art flip phone with a video camera. Before they presented it to me, the entire cast and crew recorded funny videos for me. Adam McKay proudly handed it to me.

"This is what I get for almost dying for your movie?" I joked.

Still, it meant a lot because *they* all meant a lot. I missed them after we wrapped. (Not the bear.) We created something really special. Over the years, our careers have grown and morphed in different ways—cheers to Steve Carell being famous as fuck, go Brick!—but we always stayed in touch.

After the first *Anchorman*, Paul Rudd even stayed

in my home. Rudd, his wife Julie, and their son moved into my house on the hill in Laurel Canyon because he was filming *The 40-Year-Old Virgin* with Carell, and I moved to a beautiful brownstone in Manhattan while on Broadway for *Sweet Charity*.

That how it's always been with the *Anchorman* cast. We'll always be one big, crazy, happy family.

Always.

For what it's worth, I would argue that *Wake Up, Ron Burgundy*—the uncensored, cutting-room-floor version of *Anchorman*—is even better than the original movie. It was essentially the first movie we made. That film included the amazing Alarm Clock bank robbery scene, in which I got to see Amy Poehler in action for the first time. She'd just started on *SNL,* and I remember asking Adam who this hysterical woman was. She and Maya Rudolph did a hilarious riff about the werewolf mask Maya was wearing while robbing the bank ("I am a ma'am, ma'am...How many werewolves do you see around here wearing a skirt?...None!"). It was clear Amy was going to be a star. But test audiences had wanted more of the news team and the love between Veronica and Ron, so an entire month of shooting was shelved to make what became *Anchorman*. Alas, the powers that be didn't release *Wake Up,*

Ron Burgundy theatrically—it's part of the bonus DVD, et cetera—because if they had done so, they would have had to pay us for it.

It's often forgotten that *Anchorman* wasn't a commercial success right out of the gate. When it hit screens on July 9, 2004, it was deemed a total flop. The initial weeks were tough. The first weekend numbers were disappointing enough that a friend of mine, who ran part of DreamWorks, the studio that released the movie, called me on the first Monday crying. "We flopped," he said. By its third week, it had dropped to the sixth spot.

Two years later, though, I got an enormous check from the DVD and VHS sales. Will and I always laugh that it became the gift that kept on giving. As it grew, and as generations of kids and people started to find it, it became what it is now. A smash hit. A cult classic. Grossing nearly $100 million worldwide.

We created something amazing, and then we did another one, and another.

Bing bang boom.

TWELVE
METATARSAL #5

In 2004, I flew to New York and auditioned for twelve hours for the role of Charity Hope Valentine in a Broadway revival of the Cy Coleman, Dorothy Fields, and Neil Simon musical *Sweet Charity*. This was the show that was originally directed and choreographed by none other than my hero, Bob Fosse, and when it premiered on Broadway in 1966 it had starred his then-wife, the legendary Gwen Verdon. Now there was a chance I could be Charity, too. It had been an incredible few years in my career. But this was about to be a pinnacle.

I was riding the *Anchorman* high when the chance to be in the musical came my way. It doesn't matter who you are, though—you don't just jump into that role. Charity Hope Valentine, "the girl who wanted to be loved," is a character who barely ever leaves the stage. If you're not dancing as Charity, you're dancing *and* singing. And if you're not dancing and singing, you're acting and crying and trying to make people laugh, all at the same time. It's one of the hardest roles in all of Broadway, and certainly the hardest I had ever done.

I wanted it. Dance had been my number one love, all my life, and this was my chance to do what I'd been working toward since childhood.

I started in the prestigious Julie O'Connell Dancers at age ten and danced with them for the next five or six years. We did tap, ballet, jazz—everything. If ever I was depressed, my mom would say, "When was the last time you went to class? It's been a week? That's why. You need to go."

It was the 1980s, so we wore neon unitards, leg warmers up to our thighs, headbands, and wide belts. We danced to eighties pop, some of which was pretty terrible (here's looking at you, "Neutron Dance"). Then, one day, I was walking through the Debbie Reynolds Studios in North Hollywood, where we rehearsed, when I heard a very different kind of music coming from one of the other studios: Studio F. I think it was a Melissa Etheridge song, but whatever it was, it was a siren call to me. I peeked in to watch, and my whole body froze.

What is this? I thought.

Leading the class was a dancer named Doug

Caldwell. Doug's work mixed ballet and modern, though I'm loath to use the word "modern" because that is its own thing. Doug's style was something entirely new: fluid and beautiful, with every fingertip, every part of the body, emotionally in tune. Here was a man doing something that was filled with passion and love and spirituality.

Doug had been a ballet dancer, but he didn't have the best turn-out, so he switched to choreography and teaching. It was the same story as Bob Fosse, who also had horrible turn-out. He'd pivoted to create his mind-bending dance filled with uncanny turn-in and angular poses, an art form all its own.

Doug Caldwell had invented an entirely new and beautiful form of expression, too, a place where balletic and modern met, but not flexed-foot modern. He drew gorgeous lines, which led to what was known as "the reach." Lyrical, as Doug's creation would come to be known, would eventually lead to contemporary, which is now the big thing. Back in the mid-eighties, lyrical was just getting started as a dance form all its own. I could feel the soul through every movement the dancers made, the arms reaching for something, a yearning in the body that amplified the inner yearnings we dancers so often carried.

I was hooked instantly.

I found Julie O'Connell the next day, determined

to chase this new art form. "I have to do this other thing now," I said. She understood and gave me her blessing.

I was fifteen years old.

Going to class with Doug was church for me, for all of us—eventually we'd actually call it "church." Doug's dancers stuck with him for years. We would see the young ones come in and stay, and then more young ones, and more. But there was a core group of us that had always been there, each with our own spot for his warm-ups. If anyone even put their towel down near my spot, or any of our spots, we'd pick it up and move it. *This is my spot,* I'd think. I was always to the left of the mirror, first row.

That was my spot for thirty years of dance with Doug Caldwell, from sixteen to my mid-forties. I had started dancing when I was three and have been in dance classes ever since, often for twenty-five hours a week in the summers when I wasn't acting. I loved it. It was life. I would eat a huge bowl of pasta Parmesan to get the carbs. Sometimes I'd go to work at *Married... with Children,* leave, and head straight to dance class until eleven o'clock at night. It saved me.

Some days I'd take as many as five classes: Doug's

class, Alex Magno's class, and three others. I relished Alex's technical and challenging warm-ups. He was a Brazilian dance teacher, and his class was all sensuality. When I was older, I'd act as his assistant, modeling the warm-up for everyone.

But Doug was where my heart lay. And he loved me. Once there was one perfect technician in our class—every *t* was crossed and *i* dotted. I'll always remember what Doug said about me, though, while referencing this dancing technician: "Christina is not the *best* technician, but she's the only person I want to watch in class." I still hold those words close.

I wasn't a technician and was never fully a ballerina either, but I knew how to move, and I like to think that my lines were beautiful and my reach expressive. I went to Doug's class at Studio F when I was feeling sad and wanted to be happier, or sad and wanted to be sadder, or happy and wanted to be happier. There I was able to release the pain I was feeling in my life. I was there for myself and for my heart, for my soul, for my spirit.

I did that for thirty years with this man, and with Alex.

Every movement Doug made expressed his soul, and that's what I wanted to replicate in my own dancing. He listened to every tick, every boom, every sound, every breath of the music, and danced accordingly.

There was so much crying in that class, and it was never performative, not once. It was real and true.

Some nights, after years of building a friendship, we'd go to his house after class to drink red wine and watch *So You Think You Can Dance*. Once the show was over, we would dance again for hours, even though we'd already had a three-hour class.

Doug's dance room was part of his carpeted living room, and we would freestyle and do floor work. I would sometimes look down to find that the entire top of my foot was bleeding from the carpet, but I didn't care.

I still have scars on my feet from those nights. I loved being around that bunch of dancers, around Doug. I love dancers. I love their whole world. It is my world.

Or was.

I was a damn good dancer. Damn good. I wasn't a technician, but yes, I think I could dance.

As for Doug, well, he knew chronic pain, too. When you dance all day, every day, and teach conventions all over the world, you're going to hurt everywhere. As he got older, his pain only grew.

One day I got a voicemail from him.

"Hello," he said. "I'm doing so good. Can't wait to see you. I miss you and can't wait to see Sadie."

Sadie too had loved his classes. I remember picking her up from her first lyrical class, and she said, "Mom, I know what you've been talking about, and I know what Doug has been talking about. I almost cried while I was dancing."

I texted Doug immediately: "Shit, well done."

I listened to his voicemail and made a mental note to call him. But before I got the chance, a friend texted me, "Have you talked to Doug?" After I texted no, he texted back, "He's dead."

I lost it. I didn't stop crying for a week.

I still have his last voicemail, the call I never got to return. I keep saving it so I don't lose it. But I will never return it, never tell him once again how much that reach expresses something fundamental about me, something deep in my soul that can only be touched by dance.

Dance was everything to me, and the chance to dance on Broadway? I could not let this pass me by.

Every single detail of what happened next is burned into my mind because it was the most devastating thing I've ever been through — and yes, I can say that even knowing everything *else* I've been through.

You with the Sad Eyes

It is Chicago, March 5, 2005. I have auditioned and been offered the role of a lifetime, and now I am in the Windy City preparing for previews before heading to Broadway.

It is the first night of previews. My mom has flown in, my sister, and my best friend, too. My family who live in the Midwest are all there. Before the show, I am standing onstage behind the curtain with everyone in the cast — usually we do funny things to get us loose and then circle up. This night, though, I simply say, "Guys, tonight is really important to me. My whole family is here." They understand.

Then I'm standing stage right in the wings while the cast does "Big Spender," one of the few numbers Charity Hope Valentine is not in. My job is to run out near the end and twirl around a lamppost in the center of the stage. At some point in the scene, I have to fall into a lake — which is just a big hole in the stage where the stage manager squirts me with water. I am wearing difficult, clunky shoes, not my dance shoes, because regular dance shoes would get ruined. I come back up and then go back down again, more water, back up. The secrets of live theater, folks!

I come out onto the stage to do my part, the music starts, I run to the lamppost, take a step, and my heel goes off to the side and...

SNAP!

That is a bone.

Oh my god.

I'm alone on the stage. And my first line?

"You ever have one of those days?"

I look down, and my foot is coming out of the shoe sideways. My friend Tyler Hanes, who plays Charlie, comes out and I'm dancing around him while internally flipping out. I know something is seriously wrong. Tyler pushes me into the "lake," where I find Beverly Jenkins—who is, by the way, one of the few stage managers to ever get an honorary Tony Award—waiting there with the water bottle, ready to drench me.

"Beverly, I broke my foot," I whisper. She looks aghast, squirts me nonetheless, and up I go, back onstage. Stage business ensues. Then I go back down.

"Go call an ambulance," I say.

"What?" Beverly says.

During the next scene, I do a complete song and dance number on what I would later discover to be a broken fifth metatarsal. The pain is twisting up my leg as I try not to puke. Finally, I get to the part where Charity leaves the stage for a minute. I run off and promptly faint.

In the dressing room, the EMTs want to get me out of my costume so Dylis Croman, my swing, can use it. I tell them that they can take off my wig and my shoes but not my dress, as I'd be naked, and then they blue-light me away.

April 6, 2005

How does one explain it when it feels like in a moment you lose everything? But I kept going. I can't stop now, I thought. I can't give up. Sitting in that hospital with my red dress still on, I had a moment of falling apart. A moment of, "Why the fuck did this happen to me?" Then a mode switched in. A mode that I CAN'T GIVE UP. I can do this.

Goddamn it, don't replace me.

That night, Dylis Croman did an incredible job stepping in for me. The producers wanted me off the show after that. I was devastated but not surprised—the standard healing time for a break like this is twelve weeks.

I wasn't giving up without a fight.

"I'm going to do it in six," I said.

I had to stay out of the previews for those six weeks—my understudy, the brilliant Charlotte d'Amboise, initially covered for me while we finished our out-of-town run. I did everything I could to get better faster. I would swim with my bad foot up above the water—next time you get in a pool, try to swim breaststroke with one leg held out of the water. I needed to keep my lungs going, my body fit, because it's such a challenging role. I was determined to do whatever it took, even if I had to learn to swim with one leg sticking up out of the pool.

While the previews were in Boston, I was heading to Harvard every day to use their special machines, probes, and tech. I'd meditate constantly, too, setting my intention that this bone would heal in six weeks, not twelve. Agape's Dr. Michael Beckwith, who has now been in my life for thirty-something years, said, "I need you to visualize a doctor saying, 'I've never seen a bone heal this fast before.'"

I pictured it, over and over again.

The whole time, I could feel the producers trying to push me out. They took my face off the Playbill—shit, they wouldn't even let me come to an opening night party.

The accident happened in March. Pretty soon it was Good Friday. My doctor called me.

"I've never seen a bone heal this fast before," he said.

The next call I got was about ticket sales in New York plummeting because people had heard that I might not be in the show. I was told *Sweet Charity* was shutting down.

I had just healed a bone faster than a human person should be able to heal a bone, but all the investors saw was their lost investment.

"Give me two hours," I said.

I started calling everyone, from the director of *Jaws* on down.

"I need a break," I remember telling Steven Spielberg. "In the form of half a million dollars."

Unsurprisingly, I got nowhere with anyone. Then my choreographer, Wayne Cilento—a gentle, beautiful human being—called me. "They already put the sign up backstage, Christina, telling the cast that the show's over on Sunday."

"Don't let them get other jobs," I said. "Don't."

And then I put up the $500,000 myself.

My agent said to me, "Either you're the stupidest person I've ever met or you're a fucking genius." Turns out it was a bit of both. Stupid: It was half a million bucks. Genius: The other investors realized I was serious, and by Sunday—the deeply appropriate day of the resurrection of the Lord—I got a call that confirmed we had the money we needed to continue.

That same night, the cast threw a closing party. Denis O'Hare, who played Oscar, secretly filmed me sitting there with everyone as they cried, all thinking it was over.

"Don't get another job, please," I said to everyone. I knew we were going to be safe, but I couldn't tell them yet.

"Christina," someone said, "it's *over*."

The next day—Easter Monday—we announced

that the show was back up. My foot was at 45 percent.

Now the question was, could I even do this? I was still crying in the morning because I woke up in so much pain. The investors told me they'd have Charlotte d'Amboise do the show if I couldn't prove to them that I could pull it off.

"We need you to do the whole show by yourself in a studio."

I fucking did it.

I put on my unitard and my chopped-off sweatpants and my Fosse boot with the brace inside, little wires and metal to keep the foot from moving too much, and I did it. The entire show, with someone reading the other lines—I did all my dance numbers, all my songs, in front of Wayne Cilento, the choreographer.

I'll never forget the look on his face when I finished. As he called the producers, he was crying.

"She fucking did it!" Wayne said through tears.

I sat out the show during the rest of the previews because I kept hitting my foot with my cane during "If My Friends Could See Me Now." I knew that for me to be there on opening night, I needed to skip one particularly balletic scene filled with leaps. By that time everyone in New York—even the sad little *New York Times* critic who panned me—knew about my broken foot. It was the talk of the town.

When I walked into restaurants, people didn't look at my boobies anymore.

They looked at my foot.

This was a first.

Even though Ben Brantley at the *New York Times* didn't like what I did—his comment "While she executes her steps with care and precision, dance is not a transcendent form of self-expression for Ms. Applegate" was horribly brutal about a person basically dancing on one foot—enough folks did. Even the notoriously picky Michael Riedel from the *New York Post* wrote that I was "dedicated and determined" and that "she tamed [me] with her charm, warmth, vulnerability, and expert comic timing (all this, while icing the broken foot during the intermission)."

April 2006

So I fought, and fought! I won, and I lost. So distracted. So I go to Boston, in support for me, for them. On a mission to heal in miracle time. Praying, healing, trying. But yet allowing God to do what needed to be done. Then they shut me out, my god! "The company doesn't want you here. Don't come around. Stay away from the show you started. The show that is up because of you."

Whatever. Hit me again and again. I will prevail; I will not falter. Try it!!

So "Good Friday" came along. Oh yeah, watching someone else do your show is wild... So they closed us down. Didn't cry. Got still and began the process of getting us all back together. How can I say goodbye to distraction, to all of it? How can I go back to L.A. without having finished? How can all the hard work and time and growth we put into this just fall away in one moment? Well, it only lost me a big phone bill and 500 thousand dollars. Now I do this for free. Because I love it... So now I am here watching a rehearsal without me in it. So strange. Yet it's okay now. This is work. Not about ego. It's important. I never knew I was a fighter. I am focused and driven and determined. I love who I am right now. I love you, foot. I know you are perfect. I am ready. To prevail, to succeed, to be happy. I love being here. And all is well. I've been angry, devastated, joyous, pained, remorseful, the whole nine yards.

I pushed so hard and fought so hard not because I needed to play Charity and win a prize. Instead, I had tapped into a self-protectiveness that had been slowly building within me. I had to protect twenty-six people

I loved, twenty-six people I'd just spent months rehearsing with, who were going to lose their jobs if I didn't dance.

I still had a 55 percent broken foot when we opened on Broadway. I danced with the fear of God that I could break my foot again.

My foot never quite healed correctly because I danced on it for the entire run. Back then, I displayed a grit that I sometimes worry I don't have anymore. But I've always been a survivor that way.

Playing Charity, insisting I would do so with a broken foot, and taking a significant financial risk was love made manifest. It wasn't about ego or Tonys or a better review in the *Times*; it was about keeping that cast together, keeping them in work and fulfilled, letting their genius shine onstage after all that effort. I couldn't just let it die.

I'd dance on one leg again for that kind of love.

On the morning of May 10, 2005, I was lying in my bed in my town house on Eleventh Street in Manhattan. I was living there while performing in *Sweet Charity*, and as I was luxuriating in a rare late-morning start, I got a beep on my pager. It was a message from my publicist. She had some news.

I let her words sink in. I was alone, and I didn't call

anyone. I wanted to really feel it, but I couldn't—I just couldn't be excited for myself. Part of me knew that this was the culmination of a life's dream, my Broadway dream. Another part of me heard that girl from all those years ago saying, "You're doing it." I put the leash on my dog, Tallulah, and walked north to the Fourteenth Street subway station. There I headed east on the L train and changed to the 6 train, and then up to Candle, a vegan place on the east side that I love. I got my favorite sandwich—the Cajun Seitan—and tucked it into my backpack, along with my purple hippie-dippy blanket and a book to read. Then the two of us headed farther north on the 6 to Hunter College, where I walked west into Central Park to Sheep Meadow. There I sat on my blanket with my sandwich, Tallulah staring up at me, begging for a bite.

As I was trying to not eat the entire sandwich—it had been known to revisit me while I was dancing—my phone rang. It was Michael Riedel from the *New York Post*. He would eventually write that nice notice about me, but he hadn't always been so kind. At the behest of my publicist, I took the call.

"Congratulations," he said. "How are you celebrating?"

"Well, Michael," I said, "I'm sitting in Sheep Meadow eating my favorite sandwich. And in a few minutes, I'm going to walk to Columbus Circle and get on the train and head down to the theater and do another show."

"Have you told anyone?" he said.

"Nope," I said. "I'm just sitting in the meadow with my dog and I'm having my vegan sandwich and I'm okay."

I thanked Michael for calling and hung up. I was alone again. I didn't call my mom. I didn't call my friends. I did nothing. To call them all to tell them about my Tony nomination would have counted as me "doing it," gloating, being a pill, embodying the worst of my business, and anyway, I didn't know how to feel. I wanted to hate myself because I didn't feel I deserved it. Truthfully, I have never known how to deal with the fact that I'm a successful person and yet I hate myself. That breeze called happiness seldom wafted by whatever hammock I was in, and it certainly didn't blow that morning in Central Park. All I'd ever wanted in my life was to be onstage in a Fosse-inspired show. But then Brantley had attended previews when I still had to sit out parts of the show to save myself for the actual run, and I'd danced the rest on a broken foot, so in being brutally critical he had made me feel that I just wasn't good enough.

Tallulah and I walked to the south part of the park, got on the subway at the Fifty-Ninth Street station, and headed down to Broadway. I got ready to do another show.

When I arrived, the cast and crew whooped and hollered. I looked at them, all these wonderful people.

"Let's get ready. Let's do what we have to do."

Charity was alone, but she had made it. She was okay. She did it. She danced on one foot and made something out of nothing.

THIRTEEN

KIBITZ KISMET

When I was eighteen, I took a short trip to Amsterdam when I was in the UK for *Married... with Children*. I was absolutely floored by the place and its people. The city was beautiful with its winding canals and cobblestone streets.

I wished then, and still wish, that I'd been born Dutch. One of the stereotypes about Dutch people is that they're plain-speaking, and because they "drink a lot of milk, they are therefore tall," as a Dutch man once said to me.

In the end, not being *actually* Dutch, I did the next best thing: I married a Dutchman. But it took a long time to come to fruition. Our journey has been long and cosmic and spans a couple of lifetimes. I always refer to it as Kibitz kismet.

This is why.

* * *

In the first lifetime, I met Martyn LeNoble in Los Angeles in 1994 when I was twenty-two years old. I had long realized that Duran Duran's John Taylor was not, after all, going to be my husband, but I still wondered if one day I'd marry a rock god. My first husband would turn out to *not* be a rock god, which was perhaps one of the many reasons that relationship didn't work out. Still, in my mind, I had the vision of a scruffy punk rock guy. He would always show up when I was meditating, an idle but persistent reverie I could never quite escape.

Then, in 1994, a scruffy punk rock guy appeared for real.

I was at the Kibitz Room on Fairfax. My friends and I would often head to Kibitz after going to the clubs.

As I was innocently chomping away on French fries in my booth, a guy came around the corner, and there he was, bleached blond hair, missing teeth, a brown button-down shirt over a T-shirt. My breath was taken away. *This is him,* I thought. *This is my punk rock god, my punk rock fantasy.* He was the epitome of a real kind of cool back then. If you think you're cool, you're most likely not.

Martyn LeNoble actually deserved the word.

You with the Sad Eyes

Here's this dude who has lost his teeth but doesn't even remember *how* he lost them. (Cool.) He started playing bass in a band when he was fourteen and ended up in Los Angeles playing with two of the great underground punk bands—Thelonious Monster and Too Free Stooges—and eventually cofounded the band Porno for Pyros. (Very cool.)

Our friendship began that kismet night, and he would sometimes show up at the parties I threw. At one of them, his sister noticed that she'd been ditched by her brother while he and I decamped downstairs. We spent three hours talking. We got each other. We were immediate friends.

The same night, some dude from a boy band arrived, uninvited. I remember thinking, *I'm sure you're great, but I would never invite you to one of my parties.* My friends tended to be out-of-work musicians, people who, unlike the boy in the band, know how to play music. I had Jim Morrison's piano, and bongos and conga drums and guitars, and everyone was just jamming and hootenannying. There he stood, Boy Band Boy, in his Adidas tracksuit. He turned to his two huge security guys and said, "This is what white people do."

Dude was white, too.

* * *

About a year after I first met him, Martyn fell into a dark place. One day I got a strange phone call from him and his friend, asking me to come see them. I went over to their house, and I knew immediately that something was wrong. I had to get Martyn out of there. I forced him to come with me, out to my car, and I made him sit with me and breathe. We listened to some music from the Agape church.

"Just listen," I said. "Just sit and listen."

"Get me out of here," Martyn said, referring to the house we'd just left, and the life into which he had sadly fallen.

I took him to my house to look after him. I would lie in bed with him when he was at his worst. As he tells it, by then he was in love with me. For me, it was a platonic but deeply meaningful friendship. I knew I had to do anything I could to keep him from going back to that house. I was so desperate that once in a while I'd say, "If you stay here, you can touch my boob." In my head I was thinking, *What am I doing?* But I wanted him to live—he was already so important to me. Martyn has since claimed that we kissed and that I was in love with him, too. I don't remember it like that, but okay, I'm sure it was the case.

After a week or two of this, I called his parents, whom I'd never met, and told them that I was going to fly them from Amsterdam to Los Angeles. Martyn wasn't okay, and I thought he might need them. After his parents had been in L.A. for a few days, his father took me to one side and said, "You guys fight like you're married." Later, his dad would say that in those moments, he knew we loved each other.

I still didn't know it, not truly, or at least I wouldn't admit it.

Eventually, Martyn's parents returned to the Netherlands, and Martyn felt well enough to leave. I found him back at that house. As much as I'd tried, I couldn't help him.

Our friendship, for the time being, was over.

Years later, I was shopping at Fred Segal, the now defunct but then legendary clothing store in West Hollywood, when I saw a family walking toward me. It was a tall, beautiful man and a beautiful woman, with a beautiful little girl at their heels.

It was Martyn, his then wife, and their child.

"Oh my god!" I said. "Martyn! You're alive! You look amazing. We all thought you'd be dead by now."

A day or two after the Fred Segal run-in, Martyn called me.

"I can never talk to you again," he said. "My wife said that there's too much there."

For the longest time I kept a shrine in my house, with things that I prayed for and meditated on. And part of that shrine featured a photograph of Martyn, as well as an album by Porno for Pyros. I would pray for him every day, along with all the other people I cared about.

"Okay," I said, "I understand."

It was enough that he was well and happy, or so I thought. Clearly, I was swimming up a big river in Egypt.

In the middle of 2005, my first husband and I separated. He filed for divorce at the end of that year, and soon after, I fell for a guy named Lee Grivas.

Lee was an Alaskan deep-sea fisherman, of all things—think *Deadliest Catch*—and as different from the people I usually dated as you could imagine. He was ten years younger than me and living in New York with a friend of mine when I met him. Almost instantly, he filled my life with enormous fun. He was an escape for me, especially after the end of my marriage.

At times being with Lee was like being with a toddler, right down to the making of forts in my living room (yes, we actually did that). He was an awkward guy, but he was hot and had a killer job. I loved that he didn't have anything to do with the entertainment industry. He eventually made my house in Los Angeles his home base. Every now and then he'd have to leave for a month at a time, heading off to the Bering Sea to risk his life for king cod. When he'd get back, he'd tell me all about his adventures, and the fun would return.

But Lee also had the addiction gene. He had been a heroin addict. He was off the junk when I met him, but shortly after we started dating, he picked up a pill habit, and then after a couple of years, the pills led him back to heroin. I put him in a rehab and then he went into a halfway house, but three years into our relationship, I sadly found needles in my house. My cat had tunneled into the bag and was batting at them. I just couldn't have that.

The relationship had been so fun until it wasn't. Lee was never mean. He was just young and stupid and an addict.

"You've been to enough rehabs," I told him. "I can't anymore. You have to go."

I didn't feel a thing. My wounds had scarred over, and scar tissue is stronger than any other tissue. It gives you the ability to not feel.

I moved Lee out of my house and into an apartment on St. Andrews in downtown Los Angeles. St. Andrews is famously name-checked in the Jane's Addiction song "Jane Says." Jane Bainter, the now former addict who lent her name and attendant affliction to the band, walks along the street in the song, an eerie harbinger.

We weren't talking much because it was too hard for me. I had given all of myself to try to help him, and nothing had worked. I had even talked to his mom about his problems to see if she knew something I was missing.

"I've done everything I can, too," she said. She had been through it too many times to count. "At some point you just have to let go," she said, "and you have to say, 'I can't help you anymore.'"

In late June 2008, I headed once again to Hawaii to get some relief. This time I took Martyn.

A month earlier I had walked into the children's hospital in Los Angeles, where I was volunteering to do art with the kids, and there, holding the elevator door for me, was this tanned and toned guy, smiling that toothless smile.

It had been ten years since I'd seen him last.

Martyn was at the hospital to play music for the children, and as we rode the elevator, we realized we were both wearing Converse sneakers. It felt like a Thing, more kismet. When we reached my floor I thought I'd walk away from him forever.

"Well, it was really good to see you. I'm so happy you're okay. I'm so happy."

But Martyn kept leaving me messages after that, or

calling my close friend Rachel, insisting he had to talk to me.

"Rachel," I'd say, "I don't want to talk to him. I'm fine with not talking to him."

"Christina, he *really* needs to talk to you," she'd say.

Of course I relented, and Martyn came over to my house. He wanted to make amends and say he was sorry for everything. He was sober and doing well. He was no longer with his wife.

I had a friend there that night. When he left the room, she said, "Fuck! Martyn's hot."

"Dude, go for it," I said.

"I can't," she said. "He keeps looking at *you*."

Something clicked in that moment, and I invited Martyn to come with me to the Big Island.

I hadn't officially said "Please leave me alone forever" to Lee, and he was still calling. I told a mutual friend to ask him to stop. Lee mostly left me incoherent messages.

There was one I could decipher that he left while I was in Hawaii: "Don't give up on me, Scooter." That had always been Lee's nickname for me.

It was a Sunday evening. I listened to the message, and then I put my phone down and looked out over the ocean from my hotel room. Martyn sat next to me, watching the same sunset.

I thought of Lee in that dingy apartment on St. Andrews, one of the worst places he could be. I felt guilty, and sick, in that beautiful hotel on that gorgeous island, watching the purest sun imaginable sink into the Pacific with a man I was beginning to fall in love with.

I thought too about how Lee had always said that he wasn't going to make it to his twenty-seventh birthday.

"Yes, you are!" I'd say. "You'll hold on and beat Janis Joplin and Jimi Hendrix and Jim Morrison and all the rest of them."

Three days later, while I was still in Hawaii, I got a text from a woman Lee had known in Alaska who had worked for the boat company. I had never been much of a fan of hers, so I was surprised to see her name pop up.

> Have you talked to Lee?

I texted her back.

> Why are you texting me?

She got right back to me.

> They found him.

I immediately called her.

"What are you fucking saying?" I said.

"He's gone," she said.

And I just dropped my phone.

Much later, I checked the timestamp of the message Lee had left me, asking me to not give up on him. I realized that Lee had died about one hour after he'd called me. His body wasn't found for three days.

He was twenty-six years old. He hadn't hung on after all.

I flew Lee's parents out to Los Angeles to identify his body, but because he'd vomited at the end, they weren't allowed to look at his face. The stomach acid had eaten it away in the days he'd lain there alone. Instead, they identified him by his tattoos.

This is the truth of addiction, the thing no one ever tells you until it's too late. These facts are presented here not to be gratuitous, but as a warning, as a witness, as a plea to do whatever you can to avoid this terrible fate and to help those who fall into addiction.

We held a memorial service on a yacht because Lee had always said he wanted to be buried at sea. Martyn helped with all the photo montages and everything else. I brought in all of Lee's friends from New York and rehab and his parents and anyone who knew him and loved him. It was a lot of people. He was that kind of guy.

I went into a tailspin for a long time after Lee's death.

I thought it was my fault. I still do some days. Perhaps if I'd taken his call, if I hadn't made him move to St. Andrews... So many ifs, constricting my throat, filling my heart with more self-loathing.

Though gone corporeally, Lee Grivas stayed with me for a long time in spirit.

I was haunted by him.

For the longest time, every night I would wake up at 3:15 a.m. precisely. Some nights, I'd awake to find Bella, my white cat, the one who had played with his needles, staring into the darkness with her fur up.

I could sense him too in the room.

Finally, one night I couldn't take it anymore.

"Fucking stop it, Lee. You've got to stop. I have to work. It's okay if you're here, but you've got to stop waking me up, man!"

The following night, Lee didn't show.

The day after that, a friend of mine called.

"Did Lee come to you at three fifteen as usual?" he said.

"Nope," I said, "he didn't."

"Well," my friend said, "that's probably because he came to *me*."

"Tell him to stop!" I said. Which my friend did, and Lee stopped.

Lee's mom called that same friend the next day.

"Guess who woke me up at three fifteen last night?"

I didn't understand the significance of three fifteen for the longest time. But then I stumbled upon something eerie. According to people who say they know these things, the veil between this world and elsewhere is thinnest at... you guessed it, 3:15 a.m. The barriers were down. Something impenetrable was permeable. Lee had decided to show up.

I say Lee "haunted" me, past tense, but I think he might be back.

Recently, I was reading in bed when my glasses flew off my face and right across the bed.

Am I crazy? Don't answer that! But I know it's him. Recently, I was at home getting a treatment for my pain with an acupuncturist. She taught alternative medicine at Harvard, so she's no quack—far from it.

We got to chatting, and out of nowhere she said, "Every time I walk into this room, I hear the phrase, 'To thine own self be true.'"

I almost passed out. Before Lee died, he had tattooed "To thine own self be true" across his neck.

This is not something the acupuncturist could have known. There are no photographs of that tattoo anywhere. Hell, I hadn't even *mentioned* Lee to her—why would I, when he'd been dead for nearly seventeen years by that point?

There was more.

"I can hear things," she said. "There's someone here, watching over you."

"How do you know that I know this person?" I said.

"He's giggling." I remembered all the childish fun Lee brought to my life. "And I see a bird tattoo."

That sealed it: Lee and I have the same bird tattoo.

So yes, Lee is back. He's a genial, friendly presence, and still playful. I don't mind. Sometimes I find myself saying out loud, "Come on, buddy. You've got other places to go, surely?"

But it doesn't upset me. It's fine if he wants to be here. He's a very benign ghost. He was one of the nicest guys I ever knew. There were times he could be a dick—he was a man, after all—but it's fine if he's hanging out.

I have all the time in the world.

FOURTEEN

RIGHT ACTION FOR WOMEN

I'M CURSED. IT'S A feeling I've had my entire life. Something good happens and then: boom. As I think you can tell by now, I am a big disavower of myself. I wonder how my life would have gone if that hadn't been the case. I guess I'll never know, but I like to think there's an alternate me somewhere unburdened by this self-doubt.

I feel like I'm on the edge of a cliff, about to jump into something amazing, but I never quite fall—instead, I tend to get slimed, like I'm on Nickelodeon. I think this feeling, as with so many across the years, dates back to being thirteen and my friend saying, "You're doing it." What she said changed the trajectory of my entire life, of how I view myself and process what happens to me. I'm good enough, but I'm not great.

Always, that little voice in the back of my head jeers at me, saying, "It's all going to come crashing down." As soon as I feel myself accepting goodness, I find myself pushing it away. I can't get too close to the good because when I get there, I'm going to be disappointed. That's how it feels. I've been nominated five times for an Emmy for Outstanding Lead Actress in a Comedy Series: in 2008 and again in 2009 for my role as Samantha Newly in *Samantha Who?*, and three times for my role as Jen Harding in *Dead to Me*. I've never won. I never expected to. I was complacent about the fact that I was always a bridesmaid. Fuck, though, I would have liked to win.

But this fits my soul perfectly. I have never thought I deserved anything good in any case, so not winning an Emmy is just how it is and how I expect life to go. The question of intention has, in recent years, come to haunt me. Because the universe doesn't know your intention—it only knows where your *attention* is. And where has my attention always been? The negative. Have I brought all this on myself? Have I created all of this? Have I been walking around expecting the worst all the time, only to be proven right over and over again because the universe answered my energy?

There were many times when I was getting dressed by myself and caught a glimpse of my body in the mirror, and invariably I'd hear myself complain out loud: "God, your boobs are getting saggy. I hate them."

And then I'd catch myself and say, "Don't say that. Don't say that. Don't say that." But it was too late.

I was so afraid for so many years that I would have something wrong with me: my legs, my back, anything that meant I had to stop performing, stop moving. And now here I am, forced to sit still.

Before *Dead to Me*, *Samantha Who?* was my favorite job I'd ever had. I loved being with everyone on that show. But it was hard work. I was in almost every scene, which meant I sometimes worked twenty hours a day.

The most fun nights that we ever had on that set were Fraturdays, when Fridays turned into Saturdays and on we worked. At some point during those nights, you'd see everyone from stage managers to talent carrying coffee cups, only there wasn't coffee in the cup, if you get my drift.

One week, Melissa McCarthy, Jennifer Esposito, and I were in a car being towed. We were supposed to be kind of loopy in the scene, but we barely had to act. Our sound guy, Steve Morantz, kept rolling during a turnaround, and somewhere there is footage of the three of us laughing our asses off like crazy people. I'm sure we looked like total loonies, three women stuck in a car cackling long after "Cut" was called. (We were drunk. This was not a regular occurrence, you understand, but Fraturdays could be very tough to get through.) But who doesn't want to laugh until their stomach hurts with Melissa and Jennifer? It's one of the best memories of my life.

Melissa is uncommonly funny. Her role on *Samantha Who?* sometimes felt thankless because it was small. Sometimes I'd say, "Come on, guys, give her something. You don't even know what a gem you have." One day she invited us all to see her in the Groundlings. I've never seen anything like it since. The audience was laughing so hard that sound stopped coming out of our mouths. We almost wanted it to stop so we could just catch our breath. I felt like I was going to have an aneurysm.

I remember saying to her, "When the world gets to see what you're capable of, it's over."

Cut to her shitting in a sink in *Bridesmaids*—"This sink's a goner!"—and getting an Oscar nomination for it. Told you so.

The first time I had to step back from a television show for my health was during *Samantha Who?* As early as 2001, one of my doctors noticed that there was a pattern of cancer in my family. This was before the medical profession really knew much about mutations in

BRCA1 and BRCA2, the genes that, when they work correctly, suppress tumors. When they don't work correctly, well, they don't suppress shit. My doctor insisted I start getting mammograms well before the suggested age, which back then was forty, so I started getting tested regularly.

My breasts were too dense for regular testing, and, as the doctor put it, they were also "cyst-y." He ordered up MRIs for me instead. The first one I took provided a false positive for cancer in one breast, but two months later the news was bad: the scan had indeed found cancer, this time in the other boob. There was only one option for me: a double mastectomy.

I was no stranger to cancer by that point in my life; I had lived through my mom having the disease.

> *DIAGNOSIS*
>
> *I kinda knew what the diagnosis was going to be. So much so that I put off calling the doctor back for a few days. I remember sitting in bed and making that call. "It's positive." My heart was racing, but I had no time to cry. Just immediately asked what I should do. What's the stage? Who do I call? [The doctor] kept saying, "Ductal carcinoma in situ." I think I asked her five times what the fuck she just said. In fact Rachel had to call her back a couple of times just to double-check what the*

fuck she just said. And to have her reassure me that I wasn't going to die from this. She said they remove it and you move on. Yeah, right. Regardless of what stage or nature your cancer is, you still feel frightened and feel like the walls are closing in on you. I called my mom and said I had cancer. I couldn't breathe, and when she got there, I collapsed in her lap. It was one of the few times through this process I felt mothered by her.

I immediately made changes to my life to try to get ready for whatever was to come, but whatever changes I made, I wasn't ready to face the truth. I quit smoking and went on a macrobiotic diet, but still I was told by a breast surgeon that because the cells were "microinvasive," I'd probably need a double mastectomy.

In early August, my friend Mary Kay, knowing how much I loved to keep a diary, gifted me a brand-new journal ahead of my surgery. She had intuited, rightly, that this was the beginning of a significant and potentially very painful phase of my life, and she wrote a simple but profound inscription.

Christina,

For all of your thoughts, feelings & reflections during this time. Much love.

The following are extracts from that journal, extracts that tell the tale of my lifesaving surgery. I share them with scant comment, except to say that it's poignant to me, years later, to see the tiny steps of progress—"Walked to the window," "Went all the way down to the end of the carpet"—which acted as important signposts in my recovery. I compare those achievements to how I now face MS, an illness that only ever gets worse, not better. There are no mileposts of improvement in my current situation. I have good days and bad days, but I'll never enjoy good months, good years. Those kinds of months and years are gone.

It was a hard time in my life, but I'd like to be her now, to keep her company, to borrow some of those tiny steps.

> *August 2008*
> *DAY ONE*
> *I wasn't particularly frightened the night before. At this point it's all a blur, really. But there is a "get down to business" mode I often snap into when faced with something that is beyond challenging. Went to the hospital, snuck in through the emergency room. I could feel the anxiety from everyone except me. Although I'm sure I was fucking losing it... I went to pre-op, did the basic shit. Vitals, tons of questions. Begged for something to calm*

me. Had [Dr.] Slate draw on me. All the while I was still in good spirits. Prayed… then asked for the drugs again, and my dad. And that's all I remember. The surgery was about seven hours long. An earthquake of 5.5 actually went down during my surgery, of course. Basically I felt NO pain. I was on the drip and Martyn and I watched a documentary.

DAY TWO
Barely remember. All I know is I couldn't move. I was peeing into a catheter. And I was on the drip. Still won't look under the gown.

DAY THREE
I think I sat up this day. But really more of the same. Too many visitors.

DAY FOUR
Sat up again. Sponge bath humiliation. So gassy. That was funny!! Walked to the window.

DAY FIVE
Walked the halls. Went all the way down to the end of the carpet and thought I was a major BADASS! Then I turned to go back

and started to dance and immediately had to get a wheelchair. What an asshole. The rest is foggy... Not sure if I looked [at my body] I think I did. But then of course the rumor was out and everything really exploded... Still haven't had a BM though which is really bad.

*DAY SIX
Am truly a walking fool. Discovered the dude with the sore ass [the sign on his door said "NOTHING PER ANUS" so we would walk by with random items like a pen or an apple, and wonder out loud, "Not even this?," and the other person would say, "NOTHING PER ANUS"], hospital hallway races... a lot of laughter. At this point I've looked. It's very sad... I look weird, deformed; the skin is numb, and feels totally different. Also at this point it all hits me like a ton of bricks. I still haven't stopped hurting: Lee, all of it. Sad. So sad... But I feel physically better. Stronger. I can really move my arms, sort of... can really sit up by myself. The catheter is gone as well as one of my drains. Which really weren't so bad. I guess everyone had the one thing that sticks out to them as the "scary" thing. To me it was the way I looked... But the drains didn't bother me. We called them my*

grenades. Six-shooters. I think that all of the kidding around and the laughter make this whole thing a tiny bit easier to deal with.

DAY SEVEN
Home!! I didn't want to leave because they took me off the drip and the transition to oral was challenging for me. For everyone I guess it's different. Some people just push through the discomfort. They didn't have to dance on a broken foot. Therefore, I am so damn sick of pushing through the pain... Oh, and I've been on every kind of laxative there is, with virtually no success. The perks of opiates and surgery.

DAY EIGHT (WEDNESDAY) TILL NOW, DAY FIFTEEN
Each day easier yet harder. I've gone to the bathroom. I've showered. But can't shave under my arms. I've had sex. Which surprises my comrades in boobs. I guess I'm lucky. But I think I'm just a goal setter. And I'm insanely turned on by my boyfriend and really couldn't deal. What we all want is someone who will accept us for who we are and what we have become. It's sad to hear these women talk about their boyfriends not wanting to look.

Or being single and fearful of what the next person is going to think. I'm not sure how I lucked out, but I think I have a pretty good idea. I'VE BEEN THROUGH ENOUGH!!! The universe has kicked my ass and I deserve some good. No, some fantastic! Some miracles, joy peace success elation passion and love. Because really, I couldn't take another fucking thing.

Oh, right, the boobs. So at this point, I'm pretty freaked out about tissue death and the feeling never coming back and the fact that [Dr.] Slate won't let me keep them on the small side... My back has a sharp weird pain (most likely my rib) as well as the front right underneath the expander. Yuck, I hate those things. The shape is so strange and yucky. They hurt, like as if you took a basketball and deflated it, put it under the mattress, and had [a fat person] lie on top of that. All the while trying to inflate the ball. My chest wall/ sternum is really sore and the skin feels chalky. My armpits are swollen. And part of my back is numb. Really this sucks.

But with all shitty things there is a counterpoint, an opposite. And there is where the good reveals itself. I am going to change the way young women look at breast cancer and how they can protect themselves from it. This is my charge. I have never felt so sure of anything. My whole world makes sense right now. Yes, I'm sad, yes it's uncomfortable, yes I hate it. But I have to see the blessing here. If I don't, I won't survive. If I don't I will just be one big pity party!

In 2008, when I was diagnosed, if you were a woman in a high-risk-for-cancer category, it cost upward of $3,000 to get an MRI. It was extremely expensive to get tested for BRCA. I was fortunate that I had the means to cover such costs for myself, but I knew thousands of women didn't have the same resources. A patient-relations expert at Cedar begged me to get the word out. I'm determined to do something about it.

I created a foundation called Right Action for Women, which aimed to cover the costs for such services, and in its lifetime the foundation was able to sponsor hundreds of tests.

I am extremely proud of this organization — we saved a lot of lives. It was my way of coping with how brokenhearted I was to lose my breasts. To this day, I feel emotionally and physically mangled by what I went through, but the organization mitigates the terrible loss I felt and feel. Helping others has a way of doing that.

But there are other ways I know I hurt instead of helped, both others and myself.

About a month after my surgery, I appeared on *The Oprah Winfrey Show* to talk about what I'd been through. I remember sitting onstage, all lights on me. It should have been a moment to share the truth.

"It becomes such a blessing. I talked to Melissa Etheridge [another breast cancer survivor] two days after I was diagnosed. And the first thing she said to me was, 'Christina, this is a blessing that's happened to you in your life. And right now, you get to start over, to change everything, the way that you deal with things in life, the way you react to things, fear can hurt you, stress can hurt you, this is the time that you have the opportunity to change the way you eat, everything you do.'"

Here's how I feel about that interview now: it was bullshit. Yes, Oprah was wonderful to have me on the show to promote my foundation and bring awareness to BRCA—even my amazing oncologist, Philomena McAndrew, came on. I will be eternally grateful to have had that kind of platform to help women, but I wish I'd used it differently in terms of what I said. Frankly, I was disgusted by what came out of my mouth. I had lied, thinking that I was being uplifting. I was acting like Little Ms. Warrior, but that's not how I really felt. Worse, I'm sure I was just making women who had a similar diagnosis, and who were perhaps sitting in their homes watching me on *Oprah*, feel even more devastated, even sadder because there I was, talking about fucking blessings when they were going through a living hell. I was setting up a paragon that no one going through cancer could ever rightly live up to, and for what? To show that I had somehow overcome through steel and resolve?

During that interview, I even doubled down by talking about how "they can make some very pretty boobies," comparing what I was facing after my double mastectomy with the hell my mother had gone through before me when she had been butchered by her cancer surgery years earlier. The truth was, I was alone and sad and mourning something that is the most intimate and devastating of amputations, and no amount of plastic surgery can ever make up for it.

Later, I did an interview with Robin Roberts, yet another breast cancer survivor, and once again I bullshitted my way through it, saying things like my boobs would still be sticking up when I'm dead. I was such a liar. At the end of the interview, I got up from the chair and fell against the wall, sobbing. Robin still remembers.

I recount all this to say that when I got my MS diagnosis, I was determined to do it differently. Now I'm going to always be honest. I'm not going to lie anymore. MS sucks. Every little stinking part of it sucks, not least of which, there's only downhill with MS — it's not like you can get rid of the cancer, get breast reconstruction, and move on, which was certainly how I described my journey to Oprah, Robin, and others.

I think women feel less alone, and more empowered, if someone tells them the truth. In my mind, I see a woman, whatever she's suffering from, saying to herself, "I've had a great day today, and that's so much more powerful because I've had sixteen terrible days leading up to it." This is more meaningful than telling women that they should feel like, "I can do this" *every* day or "This is a blessing." I imagine plenty of women lying in their hospital beds thinking, *I feel like shit today, but yesterday was a good day, and what's really important is that somebody* hears *me*. Surely that's how people feel less alone, rather than someone talking about blessings and pretty fake boobies. At least that's how I've felt when honesty cuts through the fake veneer of "Make the most of it" that's so often demanded of women.

Recently, I learned that my friend Clea had developed cancer. We talked on the phone about our pain and the pressure we felt as women to hide it. Our bodies had betrayed us, and it sucked. Full stop. We were on the phone for four hours, crying and laughing and trading war stories.

One day, she posted something on Instagram to the effect of, "I'm strong; I've got this."

I called her the second I saw her post.

"Nope, we're not doing this today," I said. "Do you

actually feel strong? Do you actually feel empowered? Do you want to be a poster child for this disease?" I knew the answer was no. "Take it down. We're going to rework this and I'm going to help you. And every post that you do from here on out is going to be like this: 'Chemo fucking sucked. All my hair is gone.'"

We need to stop ramming blessings down the throats of people in distress. That's not how we help people.

We help people by radical, thoughtful honesty.

I had my mastectomies during the summer, so we postponed filming for the fall premiere of *Samantha Who?* a bit. When I did my reconstructive surgeries, I was back two weeks later. I didn't tell anyone I had cancer at that point. I've been a private person all my life — until now, I guess. Bing bang boom, you're welcome.

I finally told the powers that be that I was going to buy a house on the California coast to aid my recuperation. Then, without warning, I learned we'd been canceled. We had begun by following *Dancing with the Stars,* which had given us a strong lead-in and made us the number one sitcom for a time, but during the second season we'd been moved to Thursdays after *In the Motherhood.* Our numbers plummeted.

I was devastated. I must have cried for two months. I even went on this new thing called Twitter and tried to get a "Save *Samantha Who?*" movement started, but to no avail. Frankly, I just don't think the guy who ran the studio at the time liked that it was a female-heavy show.

I loved that job. I loved those people. It was one of those rare gigs where the stars were aligned. I still stay in touch with the crew, from grips to sound people to camera operators. The day we were canceled was one of the worst days of my life, or so I thought back then.

Thank god something extraordinary was just out of sight, around a bend on that California coast.

FIFTEEN

PINCH

For all the pain of losing *Samantha Who?*, I at least had my rock god, my best friend, Martyn.

In 2009, we took a trip to Paris for some R and R after the disappointment of the cancellation. There we hung out with our friends Eva Longoria and Tony Parker, her French American basketball star husband.

One night we headed to Girafe, the ultimate Parisian high-end restaurant, with its picture-postcard view of the Eiffel Tower. Much fun was had, and much *vin blanc* was drunk, until it was decided it would be a great idea for little old me to jump on the back of Tony's Vespa for a spin around the capital — Tony was sober: trust — while the rest of our group followed in a van. Though Tony was born in Bruges, Belgium, he was raised in France, so it was nothing for him to spin across the cobbles of the 16th arrondissement like a local, taking curves at twice the recommended speed, and generally scaring the bejeezus out of me while I clung to him for dear life. It helped, I suppose, that I'd imbibed just enough *vin* and done just enough dance that I was able to sweep those turns without entirely freezing up, but by the time we arrived back at Girafe, I was probably the color of the wine: pale and entirely see-through.

Any mischievous pride Tony might have felt in my terror quickly evaporated when Martyn asked to drive the Vespa with Tony riding pillion. Being Dutch, Martyn grew up on two wheels, and by the time he and Tony returned, it was Tony's turn to look both terrified and nauseated.

As a couple, Martyn and I were having fun, two best friends creating memories. It couldn't get any better, until it most definitely did.

2010: Cinco de Mayo. If I was a Laurel Canyon baby, I like to think of my daughter, Sadie, as a Patrón baby.

That May, Martyn and I went down to our house on the shore near the coastal town of Ventura for a few days. We had gotten engaged on Valentine's Day and were heading to the coast to celebrate, among "other stuff." We were lounging in our neighbor's hot tub, *varios shots de Patrón se consumieron esa mañana*, and, thanks to the tequila, at around noon I looked at my husband and said, "Chop-chop!" It was time for "other stuff."

We had already tried to get pregnant. I was getting older, and I didn't know if it was ever going to happen. Many years earlier I had written that letter to a daughter—I just knew it would be a girl—a baby I described as being "lost in the mail." The letter read,

> *"I'm going to see you, but now's not the time.*
> *When we're ready, I'm going to see you."*

Here I was, two decades later, upstairs at my house, the swell of the Pacific at my window, the unrest of the air clattering the glass, and Martyn and I? Other-stuffing like crazy. Next thing I knew, I felt a pinch—an *actual* pinch, deep inside my body.

I swear to God, I felt it.

Then I thought, *Nah*.

"Let's do more Patrón shots!" I said, on Cinco de Mayo, aka *el día de la concepción*.

I had constant checkups because I was thirty-eight years old, and the ultrasounds showed that my daughter's head wasn't growing. Eventually, we went to see a specialist.

"Her head is indeed really, really small," he said. "I think she might have IUGR."

"Huh?" I said.

"Intrauterine growth retardation."

That's not something an expectant mother wants to hear.

"Are you doing drugs or drinking?" he asked in what I can only describe as a judgy way.

"No, I'm *pregnant,* you idiot," I said, putting aside those postcoital Patrón shots on Cinco de Mayo.

I wanted a second opinion, so I found a different doctor, who was so *un*judgy that he didn't even do a cursory examination. Instead, he stared closely at Martyn and me.

"Have you two looked in the mirror recently?"

"Huh?" I said for the second time in a week. Why do all these ob-gyns speak in riddles? And why are they all *men*?

"You both have *tiny* heads," he said. "*Very* tiny heads."

I looked at Martyn and realized in a flash that he did, indeed, have a tiny head. Martyn looked at me, and I could tell by his reaction that he'd had the same realization about me.

"Your baby is *fine,*" the doctor said, chuckling. "Now get out of my office."

I know that people who are on television are supposed to have big heads, but none of this should have been a surprise. Ben Affleck has a big head—like, *abnormally* large—and when I made *Surviving Christmas* with him, they had to put me in a certain position for the posters because his head was so much bigger than mine.

I was sufficiently comforted by this realization. My baby was healthy, and it gave me hope about the logistics of the actual confinement vis-à-vis the birth canal. Still, I was a fully hysterical pregnant person.

Even though I was so excited to be pregnant, I hated the actual feeling. I was sick for the first three months, though once the second trimester arrived, I thought I could be that person, the one who did spin classes, two hours of dance and hiked the entire Pacific Crest Trail—the whole bit. Not so fast. By the seventh month, I was sequestered at our beach house almost full-time, and the state of my lethargy could be encapsulated by the fact that one day, in the middle of a perfectly fascinating conversation, I fell asleep sitting up. I ended up bedbound and paranoid: anytime I had a twinge I would shout "Here we go, guys, she's coming!" and rush to the nearest hospital.

I remember my poor gynecologist, Dr. Rothbart, walking into the delivery room at two in the morning like a zombie.

"Can we *stop*? You're nowhere near dilated."

Finally, I showed up one too many times in the middle of the night. This time, it was well after 3 a.m., and Dr. Rothbart arrived in a ratty Rosalind Franklin University of Medicine and Science sweatshirt.

"I'm inducing," Rothbart said. "I'm sick of you." (He actually loves me.)

Thank god I'd thought to do some "gardening" ahead of time. I figured the least I could do, given how little sleep Rothbart had been getting, was offer him a pleasant experience down there, or at least a clear runway. I fear there may have been areas I couldn't reach owing to my bump. Much later, during a postpartum checkup, I apologized for my barbering. Sure enough: "Yup," Rothbart said, "it was an *interesting* choice."

Rothbart got his own back, though, in the form of Pitocin. That evil drug made the contractions so much worse. The only comfort I got came from holding a little ceramic frog from the 1940s that my mom had held when she had given birth to me. This calmed me just enough, as did the doula rubbing my feet.

At some point my dad walked in and said, "What's wrong with *you*?"

"What's *wrong* with me?" I said. "Fuck you, dude. I'm having a *baby*."

At another point Martyn and I decided we wanted a mirror to watch the birth together. The nurses found one for us, but the second we looked, we both started screaming. That was the end of the mirror experiment. (British pop star Robbie Williams once joked that witnessing his wife giving birth was like watching his favorite pub burn down.)

About eighteen hours later, our little mama came out. For the first time in my whole life, I didn't care what I looked like. I didn't care about anything. I wanted my baby on my skin. I wanted to pull her out — which I did, by the way, by her shoulders — and put her directly onto my chest. I didn't care who saw my no-nipple, scarred-up tits. Didn't care. I wanted my child's skin on my skin.

Then I noticed one of the nurses crying as she looked at my bare chest.

"Are we doing this now?" I said. "Please don't feel bad for me. We're all good here."

And we were.

Sadie is a teenager now. Every Cinco de Mayo I wish her a happy birthday, and she throws something at me. This is fair: who wants to imagine their mother saying "Chop-chop!" in a borrowed hot tub before heading upstairs?

She has genetically and otherwise adopted much of my approach to life, though. She wears T-shirts that say things like

I ♥ MILFS

I've told her she can't wear that outside our house, but I don't think she listens to me.

I've never known or felt or shared love, or *been*

loved, the way I have been since that beautiful child was born. Even though we have our ups and downs like any family, there's such an extraordinary connection between us. And I'm a damn good mom—that's really all that matters to me. Have there been times I've failed? Sure. But Sadie and I always come back from it.

The other day I was dropping her off at school when she announced, "I don't want to get out of the car."

"Why?" I said. "You can't miss school today..."

"No, Mom," she said, "it's because I'm having such a great time with you."

My love for Martyn LeNoble is cellular. In fact, the love that I have for this man is deeper than I'll ever be able to adequately convey.

He is my family. And his family is my family, too. I once went to their house in the Netherlands, and his father was blasting Elliott Smith, all by himself, cooking—he's an incredible chef.

"Do you want me to turn this down?" he shouted over the music.

"Are you kidding me?" I shouted back. "You're blasting Elliott Smith. This is my happy place in life."

I love these people.

When Martyn and I got married on February 23,

2013, in my house, it was a small group: me, my friend Rachel as my maid of honor, and Martyn's friend Vincent as his best man. My friend Kathleen McNamara, who's a minister at Agape, performed the ceremony. My mom was there, as well as Marlon, Martyn's daughter from his first marriage, and little Sadie.

I came down the stairs to the song "Save Me" by Aimee Mann.

I had suspected I could never love anyone, and yet here I was.

SIXTEEN

WHO DO I THINK I AM?

AFTER SADIE'S BIRTH I stumbled upon something that would forever change my perspective about my dad.

Paul Applegate, my paternal grandfather, had lived in Pennington, New Jersey, on a beautiful property that had rolling hills and rabbits and birds and deer and the occasional bear. Paul was a heavily tattooed steelworker who would eat bologna sandwiches with mustard and always had a frosted-glass mug in his freezer. He'd fill those mugs with cranberry juice and 7UP and share it with me — to this day I love a cranberry juice and 7UP in a frozen glass. Growing up, I thought my paternal grandfather was so kind. His house felt like family, felt like home. I loved Paul so much.

During my trips to the East Coast, in addition to

seeing my mother's family, we'd also head deeper into New Jersey to stay with Paul and his wife, Olive. Olive was not my father's mother—my actual grandmother had died mysteriously early in my father's life. Olive, whose special-needs brother lived with her and Paul, never wanted my dad around, so Bob Applegate was raised by Paul's mother, his paternal grandmother. One day, when my father was seven or eight years old (as he remembers it), Paul's mother just nonchalantly announced over the breakfast table that my father's mother had died.

As I grew older, it pained me to learn that my father hated his father: I loved Paul so. I never really understood what had happened to cause such a rift. I had heard various stories about my paternal grandmother but could never get the same story twice. My father's childhood had clearly been toxic and complicated—the casual nature of how he found out about his own mother's death was an indication of the neglect he suffered—and he had spent so much of his life in pain. He would make up memories of his early life to cope, to the point that I don't think he ever really knew *who* he was—not really. He used to say he'd never even *met* his biological mother. This was not true strictly speaking, but perhaps it was better than the reality. His grandmother told him that his mother had died in the street, beaten to death outside a bar.

My father didn't even know his own mother's

name. In 2011, my half sister would eventually get ahold of a copy of my dad's birth certificate and was able to tell him that his mother's name had been Lavina Shaw. Beyond that we didn't really know anything.

And then, as was so often the case throughout my life, a TV show changed everything.

In the summer of 2013, I was able to get my father and me some real answers. I had agreed to be part of a genealogy-based TV show called *Who Do You Think You Are?* I was determined to find out the story of his early life, and specifically what had happened to Lavina Shaw. She haunted me, just as she'd haunted my father. He could barely mention her without tears forming in his eyes, so this was an incredible opportunity to gain insight into who she was, and perhaps into who *he* was, too.

The first thing I learned in New Jersey, where they had all lived, was that my grandmother's name was indeed Lavina Victorine Shaw. She was the daughter of Ovid and Lavina Shaw, and she had a sister, Delilah. Quickly the plot thickened. With the wonderful help of a team of genealogists and historians in Trenton, New Jersey, we discovered that Lavina Victorine Shaw had never actually lived with my grandfather,

Paul Applegate. In fact, they had separated before my father was even born, and Lavina had remained at her parents' house.

Here's where the story takes a darker turn.

In 1942, my beloved grandfather Paul was accused in court documents of treating Lavina "cruelly and brutally, accusing her of immoral acts, charging her that she was guilty of adultery, by reference calling her vile and indecent names, and on various dates struck and beat her." Accordingly, Lavina left Paul, but "upon his promise to treat her properly," she returned, only to face further mistreatment.

"On or about the 13th day of May 1942, [Paul Applegate did] pack most of complainant's clothes and personal effects, and [told] her to get back to Trenton as soon as possible as the trains were still running, and why should he support her when he could get a half dozen women like her for twenty-five cents?"

When my grandmother asked Paul if he intended to provide for her and for their unborn child — my father — Paul reportedly replied, "Why should I support you or the baby? It don't belong to me."

The subsequent separation agreement nevertheless called for Paul to give Lavina fifteen dollars per week to support her and my father, but seemingly no payments were ever made. My grandmother was twenty-one years old; she had no work, and no support from my grandfather. By 1945, she and Paul were officially divorced, and full custody of my father was awarded to Lavina.

As the research deepened, I felt that sinking-pit feeling at the center of my heart. The whole thing was a damned mess and accounted for so much of my father's retreat into stories that were forever shifting. Of course that's what he did: it seemed from these documents that there had been endless turmoil at the start of his life, and when one is faced with not knowing even the basics of one's own history, it makes sense to create a narrative to fill the gaps.

I had loved my grandfather Paul, but the evidence pointed to him being a terrible man — something about the phrases "Why should he support her when he could get a half dozen women like her for twenty-five cents?" and "Why should I support you or the baby? It don't belong to me." Even that chilling reference to the trains still running in Trenton. His words rang true in their specificity, and each statement was chilling in its own way, revealing cruelty and dismissal in equal measure. And to think that my grandfather had said to a court, stated clearly in the public record, that he was not my father's real father... It was hard for me to even think about. How was I going to tell my father?

Lavina, my father's mother, was not without blame

either. A doctor's note dated May 1945 was painful to read even almost seven decades later. In it, it was reported that when my father was still in his mother's care, he was treated for both pneumonia and malnutrition. I couldn't get this image out of my head: my poor father not just hungry, as I imagine many children were by war's end, but hungry to the point of malnutrition? It was one thing to come out of a chaotic family; it was another to be the victim of what can only be described as child abuse. Neither of my paternal grandparents came out of this research with much credit, and my poor father? I shuddered to think what else he'd been through as a child.

By later in 1945, Paul had further accused Lavina of adultery—which was still illegal at the time—and had both her and her supposed partner, Michael Constant, arrested. Paul and Lavina continued to accuse each other of drunkenness, too—clearly their union was beyond toxic and severely undermined by substance abuse.

With custody of my father awarded to Lavina, that's where the paper trail, at least with regard to my father's parents as a couple, ends. Lavina's mother would help with raising my father, but she died in 1946, which was probably the reason my father was subsequently raised by his *paternal* grandmother.

Then in 1955 the story comes back online. According to documents we found, Lavina died at age thirty-three, "at home after a short illness." By then she was Lavina *Walton,* and her death certificate listed her cause of death as "pulmonary tuberculosis with effusion, cirrhosis of the liver," brought on by "acute alcoholism and nutritional anemia." She was buried at Riverview Cemetery in Trenton.

Perhaps what Paul had accused her of had some validity. Perhaps her accusations about him had also been true. Either way, my father was born into an abject mess of a family, one in which his father was absent for much of his life. My dad would return to live with Paul Applegate when he was fourteen years old, though there is no record of how a man who denied his paternity treated him. My father's birth mother had been an alcoholic who neglected to feed him. His stepmother had wanted nothing to do with him. His paternal grandmother had been flippant and cruel about his mother's demise. What kind of life must this have been for Bob Applegate?

Did this unfolding and harrowing story of Paul and Lavina begin to explain a little of why my father had behaved the way he had with his own fledgling family? He was born into profound trauma; the scant stability he had known had been forged out of a dysfunctional, violent background, one dogged by abuse and alcohol. And then, out of seemingly nowhere and still at a young age, he found himself living in California, married, and a new father. What came next can never really be rationalized or explained away, and there are still times when the pain of what he did to me stops my breath. But knowing where he came from, at least, gave some meaningful context to the decisions he had made about my mother and me.

Perhaps worst of all, my father had been forced to create entire narratives from the few facts he had, stories about him not even knowing his mother, or about her being beaten to death outside a bar, or, as he says at the start of the documentary before we began the research, a story that his mother had died when he was "seven or eight years old." The truth was, she'd actually helped raise him. She'd died much later, when he was fourteen, and there was no evidence of a violent death. Can you imagine being in so much pain, having suffered so much trauma, that you misremember the fundamental details of your mother's, and your own, life? His hurt mind had scrubbed her from his past altogether. It's extraordinary what pain will do to recollections. I bear this in mind as I write this book.

I watch the documentary now and I see how flummoxed my father was, so knocked sideways by what we learned about his mother. It was as if we were describing someone else's life, as though the coordinates of his existence had been written down wrong from the very start. He believed these imagined narratives so fully that I'm sure he would have passed a lie detector test. How does one person get so unbridled from a basic truth?

We are all the products of stories we tell about ourselves, stories pieced together from what we know is true and often from stories we wish were true, and of course the ones we wish weren't. Merely in the writing of this book, I have had to assess which parts of my life are factual and which are accretions of stories that have fossilized in my life to create something cogent, when in fact each moment we live does not necessarily cohere with the next. We are so used to believing that our life story is a narrative penned by a cosmic screenwriter who has storyboarded out an entire set of episodes, seven perfect seasons culminating in an incredible finale, when in fact our lives are often just a scatter of scenes that barely hold together.

Sometimes when I read back through my diaries I feel a concussion when contemporary facts, jotted down years ago with no agenda back then other than to put them to paper, barely line up with the stories I share with friends in my day-to-day recounting of my history. It's not just a change in perspective; it's actual facts that simply don't resemble the arc of the story I tell myself. It's as if halfway through the pilot a new character shows up who is forgotten by episode 2. I'm not sure anyone has a lock on their past; no one has an ironclad memory, let alone a willingness to always face the full truth of who they are and what they did. So why should my father be any different? If he was still alive, I might have sat with him, reading these pages. It wouldn't have surprised me to hear him say that what I wrote bore no resemblance to his truth whatsoever. But this is my truth, or what I've meticulously mapped from a lesion-ridden brain and a much more reliable written historical record. Our discontinuity might have been a problem I would have had to deal with; alas, that problem is no longer mine, nor his.

What I'm trying to say is, everything's a story, everyone a tale told. My father is no different: he had taken what Wallace Stevens calls the "flickings from finikin to fine finikin" of his life, the little hints and half-truths and bald lies and everything in between, and created an entire world out of what were, essentially, whispers. And then, when I came along, those small truths and half-truths and lies had somehow coalesced into a justification for him to flee his family and move to Big Sur and raise a completely different family with an entirely new wife.

But somehow, working with him on that documentary, and hearing the entire sordid tale of Paul and Lavina, only served to deepen the love and understanding I had for my father. I may have wanted him to be someone else, my mother may have wanted the same, and I may have felt great pain and frustration that he constantly seemed to want to tell the various tales he'd created about himself as I grew up. But given what he'd been through at such a young age, and putting aside as hard as I can the abandonment that I'd always felt lay at the heart of our relationship, it was nevertheless an extraordinary and beautiful effort of love for him to come back fully into my life when my daughter was born. He was the best possible grandfather to Sadie, even if he had been at times a distant figure to me. We can only make ourselves better than where we came from. When given the chance, we can only upgrade our love until it resembles something magical and beautiful. No one can really ask any more than that of anyone.

And that's what my father was able to do with Sadie.

For all the pain my relationship with my father has caused me, the love and the need for him is undeniable. There, in my diary, right after my double mastectomy in 2008, thirty-six years after he left me, an innocent entry jumps out at me like a bright, loving light: "Went to the hospital, snuck in through the emergency room. I could feel the anxiety from everyone except me... Begged for something to calm me... then asked for the drugs again, and my dad."

* * *

In the documentary, my father not unreasonably asked me if there was any *good* news about his background, given that I'd just informed him of the sordid back-and-forth of his parents as documented in the deepest recesses of a New Jersey records office. And I found that I was able to say this, and mean every word:

"The beauty of this is that you can be incredibly proud that you broke the pattern and that you raised all of us to have strength and intelligence and talent and fight in us. And you did that with no help from anyone, Dad. And that's pretty amazing."

"That's good enough for me," he said, choking back tears. I had dropped all this information on him, a camera crew pointing their lenses directly at him. And he'd had the good grace to bear it all, and to respond with compassion to his own life after years of mythmaking.

Working on the documentary had brought back memories of wonderful times with my dad, too. We'd go camping in his white VW bus with the pop-top. Whenever he could pull over at a beach we'd do so, barbecuing and sleeping under the stars. And I loved the way he was always so proud of me.

We all might hope for some great coming to terms with those who've wronged us, in which the things we say and do heal forever the wounds we've inflicted, or the wounds we've endured. But in the end, it might just be recognizing that someone did something righteous and loving in spite of having scant modeling to draw upon that is enough. Perhaps after everything, that is the legacy and epitaph my father deserves. Born into a country coming out of a terrible war, to two people in a highly tempestuous relationship; born into poverty and anger, accusations and alcohol...given all that, the fact that I grieve him so deeply means something.

I sit on my bed and watch TV, or a friend comes over to visit, or my daughter comes home from school, or I get a text or see a funny Instagram reel, or I sit on my porch and hear the trilling house finches frantic in their attempts to raise a brood of their own, or I'm simply lighting a cigarette, and as the flame of the lighter erupts, there it is: the loss of him, as bright as the orange flame in my hand. It strikes like an earthquake, the building shaking, the flame held still, as though I can't remember what to do with it, the cigarette slowly dropping to the floor, me holding on for dear life, unable for a second to breathe or think or cry or shout or do anything approaching a normal response, in agony at the loss of a man who shares my last name, who gave me the name the world knows me by, whose twinkling eyes I can see when I close my own.

* * *

At Riverview Cemetery we discovered that Lavina didn't even have a headstone, but she had left something so much more tangible, so powerful it took my breath away: she had asked that her son be buried with her.

A few months later, my father and I were able to erect a stone. It reads:

DELILAH SHAW	LAVINA SHAW	OVID SHAW
NOV. 25, 1925	OCT. 9, 1921	SEPT. 26, 1878
SEPT. 29, 1953	MAR. 31, 1955	FEB. 13, 1950

Mom, I found you

Despite everything Lavina had been through, she had thought to keep a space for her son for eternity, a fact that moved my dad immensely. In the end, even though my father had been given so little to work with, he still managed to create so much.

My dad was nothing short of a miracle.

The key to life is forgiveness. My father had to learn to forgive his parents, just as I had learned to forgive mine, just as I pray Sadie will one day forgive me for my failings.

It's all we've got.

After my father's death in 2025, I had to come to terms with the fact that he didn't leave *me*. He didn't even leave my *mom*. He left a *business*—the music business, which might've been killing him—for something simpler, something in nature, something beautiful, and focused instead on simplicity and gardening and mountains and beaches. That's what Big Sur, and eventually up in the north of California, was for him. This I can understand. So, I love you, Dad, and I'm glad I got to have you for as long as I did.

SEVENTEEN

DEAD TO ME

In 2015, I shot *Bad Moms* with Mila Kunis, Kristen Bell, Kathryn Hahn, Annie Mumolo, and Jada Pinkett Smith. Originally, I had wanted the role of Carla, eventually played by Kathryn Hahn. When I asked the directors why they hadn't given me the part, they told me I was the only one who had scared everyone. I was given the role of Gwendolyn James, who's the worst mom, until she isn't.

During postproduction, after the movie was filmed, I went into a studio to rerecord some lines. I watched myself on the screen, matching my words to what was already taped. At one point, they paused the film. You know that moment when you pause *Love Island* or *Real Housewives* on your Apple TV to go to the bathroom and the person's face is contorted in such a way that makes them look absolutely awful? Now imagine it's *your* face. *I look so old,* I thought, trying not to freak out. I made a comment about it, and to my horror, one of the directors admitted that the studio had already asked postproduction to fix my face.

"We had to spend thirty thousand dollars to make you look younger," he said.

This business is brutal.

Until it's magic.

My job as an actor opened so many wonderful doors for me. I know how lucky I was, and I have so many incredible memories of the movies I made, the TV shows I starred in, and the ancillary work: the talk shows, the appearances on red carpets, hosting *SNL*—the list is long, and these days, sitting alone in my bedroom, I do my best not to turn these memories into statues of myself.

I got to host *SNL* twice. The first time, way back in 1993, at the height of *Married...with Children,* I was lucky enough to be in a sketch during which the incredible Chris Farley debuted perhaps his most famous character, the motivational speaker Matt Foley, who lived in his van, "down by the river." The character has long since passed into the folklore of the show, not to mention into American comedy history, and it was an extraordinary privilege to be brought so close to pure comic genius as Matt Foley debuted in the world. The way Chris planted his legs wide, continually twisting his not inconsiderable weight from side to side and forward and backward; played with a belt he could barely find; and delivered his lines with an almost manic verbal energy—it was everything a very young David Spade and I could do to not completely lose it.

If you watch closely, Spade starts to crack almost immediately, and I try to hide my laughter behind my hair, which was conveniently falling across my face. Even my hair couldn't save me when "Matt Foley" says, "I am thirty-five years old, I am divorced, and I live… in *a van, down by the river.*" That was it—I brought my left hand up to my face in a vain attempt to stifle my giggles. By the time Chris is telling Phil Hartman he wishes he could shut his "big yapper," followed by further unsuccessful attempts to pull his pants up higher, David and I were done. I think David had given up trying to not laugh out loud. I was still playing with my hair and trying to hide my face, and though I was supposed to be scowling the way Kelly Bundy might, it was impossible. Chris was now towering over me, and I was proud that I was able to tell him, without entirely breaking, that I too wanted to live in a van down by the river.

I thought I'd gotten away with it. But then Farley started to swing those big arms, and once again David and I were toast. It didn't help that we hadn't been told that Chris was about to dive full length into the coffee table, smashing it to pieces.

The sketch aired on May 8, 1993. My second time hosting was nearly a decade later, on October 13, 2012. This time I was delighted to be part of "The Californians," taking the role of Fred Armisen's fiancée, Brie, after his first wife, Karina, played by Kristen Wiig, had "died." (Kristen had left *SNL* the previous season.) Mastering that Californian accent wasn't much of a stretch for a woman who'd grown up "east of the 405."

I was also invited to create a sketch based on my former dance teacher, Madilyn Clark.

Madilyn, who sadly died in 2023, was very Fosse, and when she taught us—even when we were little kids just starting out—she would eschew using counts in favor of a kind of scat jazz. We called the fake studio Jillian Chizz Dance Studio because "chizz" was the kind of thing Madilyn would say. I got to both honor and parody Ms. Clark with my "kadonk"s, "kadunk"s, and "za-za"s—*that* is Fosse, as "Jillian Chizz" tells the bemused wannabe dancers.

At the start of the show, I'd sung my monologue, which was both nerve-racking and great fun, and the show ended with me shouting "Sadie Grace, you're the light of my life!" during the good nights. She was approaching two years old then.

In between my *SNL* duties, I'd made two appearances a year apart on *Friends:* "The One with Rachel's Other Sister," which aired in 2002, during the show's penultimate season, and "The One Where Rachel's Sister Babysits," which aired in October the following year.

I feel like a total schmuck saying this, but I'd never watched *Friends* before appearing on the show. I really didn't know much about it. I wasn't trying to be cool by avoiding it. Back then, before DVRs and TiVos, *Friends* was the ultimate in appointment TV, meaning if you were working in the evenings, as I often was, you missed it. Now, in the age of streaming, I've watched every single episode.

I played the dreadful Amy Green, Rachel's sister. I already knew Jen Aniston and Courteney Cox and Lisa Kudrow a bit socially, as well as David Schwimmer, and Matt LeBlanc and I had worked together on *Married...with Children.* He had played one of my boyfriends, from which he'd scored a brief spin-off, *Top of the Heap,* playing a very early version of Joey Tribbiani. And then there was Matty.

Matthew Perry always maintained that working on *Friends* was like being part of a lovely and loving family, and I saw firsthand how genuine that love was. I felt safe on that set, and I think that showed in what I was able to bring to the ensemble. I got Outstanding Guest Actress in a Comedy Series Emmy nominations for both appearances and won for "The One with Rachel's Other Sister."

I'd known Matty the longest. In fact, we'd known each other since we were kids working on *Charles in Charge* two decades earlier. Much later, we also made a terrible TV movie together called *Dance 'Til Dawn*.

Later still, we performed together at a fundraiser, raising money to bring Shakespeare to children in Los Angeles. Poor Matty was so freaked out beforehand—"I have to be good, I have to be good," he kept saying. I took him outside the theater for a pep talk, or as close to one as this snarky blonde gets.

"Matty," I said, "Shakespeare rolls over in his grave every time we do this. So don't stress. Seriously. Sure, you're doing Shakespeare with some of the most famous, lauded, award-winning superstars to ever live: Anthony Hopkins, Kenneth Branagh, Tom Hanks, Rita Wilson, Robin Williams. Marty Short will probably improv his way through it as usual, and stars like Smokey Robinson and Bette Midler sometimes show up. I realize it can be as intimidating as fuck to walk into that kind of crowd. But everyone's going to screw up. The audience loves it when we do. So don't worry."

I don't think my little pep talk, filled as it was with bold-faced names, helped him all that much.

A bunch of us had been doing this fundraiser for years. I was asked back every year, becoming part of what I suppose was kind of a little repertory group, comprising me, Marty, Tom and Rita, Jason Alexander, and William Shatner. Ahead of time we would do table reads where we'd always have fun, no stress, and then we'd stage an entire play, usually a comedy, with scenery and costumes, all while carrying sides. We were expected to know at least some of the lines, but it always went off the rails in the most delightful of ways.

At various breaks during the Shakespeare performances, we'd have a musician sing something, which was very true to the original staging of the plays, when troubadours would serenade theatergoers in England. We were lucky to have had Natalie Cole, Smokey Robinson, Faith Hill, and Tim McGraw.

Then one year Sir Paul McCartney showed up to provide the musical interludes.

During the rehearsal that week, when Sir Paul stepped forward to do his part, we all videotaped him — I still have video of all of us with our smartphones held up, filming each other, all of us just losing it. He sang everything you would hope for: "Hey Jude," "Lucy in the Sky with Diamonds" — you name it.

The director also gave him a couple of scenes to act in, one of which featured just me and him onstage. I can't even remember what play we were doing — it might have been *The Two Gentlemen of Verona* — but beforehand, the director secretly took me to one side.

"I want you to do something," he said, "and we're not telling Paul. In fact, we're not telling anyone. Got it?"

That's how I came to randomly plant a massive smackeroo of a kiss on his famous-Beatle face. In the lead-up, in my head I'd been saying, *Kiss the Beatle, kiss the Beatle.*

The crowd went berserk.

Paul was shocked. He said "Christina, my wife is in the front row," though I think he knew what a *moment* it was.

"I don't care," I said, and carried on with the scene.

Good things have happened to me, so, so many, including kissing one-quarter of John, Paul, George, and Ringo.

Then one year during the Shakespeare Festival I finally got to play a part I'd wanted since I was ten. I'd wanted to take the role of Maria in *Twelfth Night* because she's dirty and naughty. It was one of my happiest moments onstage.

I had always wanted to be taken seriously, even in comedic roles — see my diary from January 1988:

> *I'll show these fuckers that I ain't no comedy bullshit actress.*

The role I had been looking for my whole life was that of Jen Harding in *Dead to Me*. It was the greatest job I ever had because it was an incredible amalgamation of comedy and drama. You can't have comedy without drama, and you can't have drama without comedy — otherwise it's self-indulgent. But Jen was all of the above and more and in between. Sadly, it would be my last job.

Maybe...

Dead to Me is the best work I've ever done in my entire life — there, I said it. And you know I don't feel comfortable talking about my achievements ("You're doing it"). But the truth is, I'd been waiting for this kind of character, this moment, all my life.

Dead to Me is about two friends, Jen and Judy, who initially meet in a grief group and whose lives become inexorably intertwined. It features a brilliant script, and an amazing cast. It was an entirely female-run show, made up of whip-smart women who were kind and loving and supportive. Even before my diagnosis, the set was a place of succor. And with Linda Cardellini, I wasn't just playing opposite an astonishing actor: I was playing opposite someone I loved dearly.

Ill or not, I'm never going to have an actress in front of me like Linda ever again. She's unbelievable. She made it easy for me to inhabit the role of Jen Harding. My secret was that I didn't prep anything. I didn't want to have a plan. I simply let it happen, like I learned to do on the *Anchorman* set. I wanted to sit across from Linda and react to whatever she was throwing at me. In turn, I quipped back at her until we were playing verbal ping-pong. I think that's why the show felt so fresh. I was allowing the character to live through me, so much so that I wouldn't even memorize the lines until I got into the makeup chair each morning. I'm lucky that I have a knack for it, which comes from years of vaudeville, as I like to call sitcom work. On sitcoms, the writers sometimes rewrite right in front of the audience, and you learn everything on the spot.

With Linda, I'm not just talking about her talent, which is off the charts. I'm really talking about the human being behind all of it, and the support that we created for each other.

That support and love began immediately. She and I met for lunch one day, and the next thing we knew, we were shooting — no rehearsals. The words came out of our mouths so organically and beautifully, like it was meant to be.

But again, it was the off-camera things that really cemented our friendship. At one point she had some stuff going on in her life — as we all do — and I told her to go home and work it out. That's usually never an option, but on this set it was.

Do I need to tell you again that it was run by women?

When I first got sick, I missed two months. It didn't matter. There was an intrinsic understanding that humanity comes above work, which is rare, especially given how much money is involved.

Sets on TV shows can be brutal places.

When I made *Samantha Who?*, the days were eighteen hours long because of the camera setup: master, medium over the shoulder, medium close-up, close-up. This was the textbook, old-school way to shoot TV, which was how it went basically until *Modern Family*, when everything changed to handheld cameras. With handheld, the industry realized you could fit a twelve- or sixteen- or even eighteen-hour day of shooting with four different cameras into five hours. *The Office* and *Parks and Rec* followed suit.

On the set of *Samantha Who?*, before the turn to handheld, I'd get so upset when we would have crew members driving home on the freeway at three and four o'clock in the morning on a Friday night. I didn't have the balls to say anything about it until I made *Dead to Me*. But one night I found myself announcing, "Guess what we're doing? We're stopping work right now. Thank you," and I did an about-face and walked off the set. I was not going to risk my colleagues getting into a car accident late at night anymore.

After I got sick, we could work only twelve-hour days anyway. I think they were all secretly happy about it — not the sickness, of course, but the time. For those of us used to endless days and nights, twelve hours was a picnic. No forced calls, when you have less than the mandatory twelve-hour turnaround, which includes drive time, from the time you wrap to the time you are due back at set. No late nights. My goal in life was to be so famous and successful that I could get "portal to portal." Johnny Depp has portal to portal, which means his wrap time starts from the moment he gets home, not the moment he leaves. A rare perk.

Right before I got diagnosed, I was at the Golden Globes for my nomination for the second season of *Dead to Me*. I happened to be coming out of a bathroom when I noticed Meryl Streep and Helen Mirren walking hand in hand down the corridor. Helen stopped me, grabbed my hand, and looked me dead in the eyes.

"You are one of the best actresses I've ever seen," she said.

Helen fucking Mirren.

I didn't get the Golden Globe, but I took home Helen Mirren's praise that night. I'd like to have her words tattooed on my ass one day. (There's room.)

A few weeks later, just after we'd begun shooting the third season of *Dead to Me*, my doctor asked to talk to me on Zoom. I'd been having some numbness in my peripherals for a while, and I'd taken a raft of tests to try to get to the bottom of it. That day, I'd been asked by the director to stay at work to shoot one more scene, but I'd demurred—something I seldom ever did. I knew this call was going to be important. Maybe I already sensed how important, so rare was it for me to push back when someone wanted me to keep working.

It was a Monday at 7 p.m. My neurologist's face appeared as we connected. He looked forlorn.

"I'm sorry," he said.

Something clicked off in my head. All emotions short-circuited. I went numb, completely numb.

"I want to show you pictures of your brain," he continued.

To this day, his words reverberate in my head and my heart, my soul, my stomach, my solar plexus—everywhere.

"Here are the lesions," he said. "There are about thirty."

Most people will have maybe a couple on their spine. I have none on my spine, but more than thirty on my brain.

"What are you saying to me?" I said.

"You have multiple sclerosis."

I didn't cry. Instead, in shock, I said, "Okay, thank you very much." I closed the laptop.

I've said elsewhere that dread things follow dream things in my life. I should have called this chapter "From Helen Mirren to Thirty Lesions."

* * *

I texted the creator of the show, Liz Feldman; our unit production manager; and the producers.

"Guys," I typed, "we have an answer to why I've been having trouble on set. It's MS."

The initial sorrow and sympathy were immediately followed by them shutting the shooting week down. That was so hard for me to hear. I had always prided myself on being a workhorse.

"No, we keep going. We keep working," I texted.

"Absolutely fucking not," someone wrote. "You're not coming to work tomorrow, if ever again if you don't need it."

Everyone was ordered to take a month off so that I could figure out what the fuck was going on with my life. I don't think any other set of TV professionals would have done that. It was the most incredible group of humans. They realized it was just a TV show, something many of us might say, but which so few of us in the business ever truly believe. But they believed it, and it made all the difference.

I'd been told that my numbness was probably just peripheral neuropathy, which is a manageable condition. The real signpost of trouble had been a nerve test I'd passed. I mistakenly thought this was good news, but passing the nerve test is not a good thing. It means that there's no damage to the nerves—duh—and that the numbness is coming from somewhere else.

After that nerve test, I think my neurosurgeon knew, but he hadn't said anything except that he wanted to run some more tests to "rule some things out," hence the MRI results he shared with me on Zoom. Looking back, I know he knew. Even my chiropractor, Dr. John, knew.

I remember asking Dr. John, "Why are my toes twitching like that?"

I'll never forget the look he gave me.

"My mom has that," he said before quickly changing the subject. "Let's work on some other stuff."

We were about a month into shooting the third and final season of *Dead to Me* when I got the diagnosis. For the next few months, we all learned together how much I could do, how much I could take emotionally, spiritually, physically—all the things. My neurosurgeon wrote a letter to the producers saying that I could work only twelve hours per day, which was less than I'd ever worked in my whole life.

"If she says she needs time, you have to give her fifteen minutes," the letter said. Sometimes I would take those fifteen minutes to go to my trailer and put my feet up, take some pain meds, cry, scream, not always in that order.

The pain I felt initially was not like it is these days: back then, it was more of an I-have-no-strength kind of pain, rather than the often excruciating agony I'm in now. I had always danced through pain and was able to do so on *Dead to Me* to complete the season.

The filming schedule for the last season was supposed to be only ten weeks, shooting about an episode a week. If you've seen the show, you might imagine that the scripts for that season were changed because of my diagnosis, but the truth is, those scripts were written a year before I got sick. Not a word was changed—the only thing that was changed was the blocking to lessen how much I had to walk in each scene.

We started in the summer of 2021 because James Marsden, the movie star that he is, was needed on a different project. We had to shoot the fugly twat's scenes first for a month. (I adore this man—he knows he's hot, I know he's hot, everyone knows he's hot.) Accordingly, we were shooting totally out of order, and in the end, the final season took just shy of a full year to complete.

There were some days I simply couldn't make it to set. I remember trying to get down the stairs of my house at six o'clock in the morning, and I could make it to only the ninth stair. I know exactly how many stairs there are—six and then nine, and then two more—and I couldn't make it any farther. I fell to the floor, dropped my bags, and waited.

I sat on that ninth stair for a while, my driver outside, but eventually I called Joe Hardesty, one of our co-executive producers and one of the loveliest people I've ever known.

"I can't come," I said to Joe. It broke me—me, the good kid who never missed a day of work in her entire life, the good girl who listened, kind to everyone, never complained, on time, and who didn't bring her shit to work. So much so that one day years earlier, while working on *Married... with Children,* I called my then agent and told her I was suffering from crippling menstrual cramps. She, in turn, called my manager to say, and I quote, "I don't think Christina's fit to work right now because of her mental state." So much for female solidarity. I went to work anyway, because there was nothing wrong with my mind. I wasn't drooling over my sorrows or talking about my difficult childhood—it was just that my uterus was on fire.

* * *

Eventually, my disability was showing up so much on camera that Netflix wondered if perhaps we needed to shut the show down—they could see my pain in the dailies and didn't want to torture me. Even Liz Feldman suggested we end early, so understanding was she, as were the rest of the crew and cast.

"We can wrap up what we've done already," she said, trying to save me from further agonies.

"No, fuck no," I said. "We have a story to tell. We have an obligation to these two characters."

I meant it. To me, Judy Hale and Jen Harding, the two people Linda and I embodied, were very much alive. I believed we had an obligation to finish their story.

So that's what we did.

By the end of making *Dead to Me*, I had to have three people help me down the stairs of my trailer to get to my wheelchair to even get to set. I was completely stripped of my independence, my autonomy. Linda would say to me, "Whatever you want to do, I'm good. I love you. It's more about you and your life and your health than everything else."

I was dead set, though. "No, I'm finishing this." I danced through the pain, and when I was done, I collapsed, and it was 2022, and I've been collapsing ever since.

On our last night of filming, Linda and I shared an incredibly emotional scene. Liz Feldman kept stopping us and saying, "Can you guys stop crying so much? It's really not helping the scene."

We were sitting in bed together. Linda says,

—I've had the best time, Jen.

I misunderstand her and think she's talking about Mexico, where we are.

—Me too.

But she corrects me.

—I mean, I've had the best time... with you.

—Me too.

I don't think either of us was acting then.

On every take, when she spoke, my whole stomach lurched because I knew it was our last moment together, and we'd been through so much.

I think this was the first time in my life that people saw I was good at what I can do.

And it was all being taken away.

I don't like not finishing things. That's another reason this illness has been so brutal. When I got sick, I realized quickly that my career was finished, and so prematurely. It's not just having an illness that makes work impossible; it's everything that goes into making movies and TV shows. I can't get up at five thirty in the morning, can't sit in a car for long periods on the way to set, can't bear people touching my face. I just can't do it anymore.

The last time I truly felt a part of Hollywood was at the 75th Emmy Awards, when I was nominated for Best Supporting Actress in a Comedy Series for my role in *Dead to Me*. I took Sadie as my date. I don't think I would have made it through without her by my side—mostly because she forced me to stay so she could see all her favorite people on stage. Cough, Natasha Lyonne, cough.

I was terrified that night. It wasn't my first time in public with my disease, but it was my first time in a room full of my peers. I was so scared, and I was the first presenter of the whole show.

My dress was heavy, and I grabbed the arm of my pal Anthony Anderson to stabilize me. As I walked out, every single person in that room stood up.

It was something I'd always dreamed of, walking onto a stage and having people stand up and clap for me. But in that moment, I kept thinking, *They're standing up because I'm sick. They're standing up because I'm sick and not because they appreciate all the work I've done*. That's why I made a joke. I wanted everyone to know that it was okay, they didn't have to feel sorry for me. Even in a room full of my peers giving me a standing ovation I couldn't accept their approval.

I started to cry.

No one had ever stood up for me for my acting before, and here they all were. *Christina, look at everyone and see that this is a moment and they are all loving on you.* It was hard for me to accept it, but I hold on to it so dearly in my heart. *Thank you.*

But then, they stood up for the next person, and the next person, and the next. Up and down and up and down. Sadie and I couldn't keep it together. We were doubled over laughing.

"I thought it was just for me!" I said, as we all stood up yet again. "Guys, come on. I thought I had a moment, you assholes!" Eventually, after the millionth standing ovation, we just sat in our seats, too tired to get up again, losing our shit giggling at the ridiculousness of it all.

I didn't end up winning the Emmy that night, but it was still a special evening. Regardless of my self-deprecating nature, I know deep down that it was all love and appreciation. In a room filled with some of the best, most talented people I've come across in my five-decade long career, I felt their warmth in my heart, even if I have to fight my inner critic to fully embrace it. It's a moment I will forever be grateful for from my peers. One that plays over and over again in my mind.

Sometimes my daughter's friends tell her, "Oh my god, your mom, your mom!" It fills me with that familiar shame. I still hear those words, "You're doing it," echoing endlessly.

But then, recently, my daughter said, "You are the best actress I've ever seen."

She's the person I love most in this world, and I think maybe, just maybe, her voice echoes the loudest.

EIGHTEEN

THE LADY IN THE BATHTUB FROM *THE SHINING*

"What's my Hawaiian name?" I was in Hawaii with my friend Shaney Boy.

"Kilikina," he said, Kiki for short. To this day, no one on Hawaii calls me Christina.

I'm Kiki.

Kiki is my real name. Kiki is who I really am. She's fierce, and free, and she doesn't have MS or trauma or low self-esteem or a history of bad decisions.

She's a simple, sweet, sharp, smart-mouthed dancer. Kiki is both who I could have been, and who I really am.

When I first visited, I met a woman who had just had her first child, Pua. Back then, I felt a kinship with Pua, and as I watched her grow, I was so happy that she had no inkling that I was a TV star back in the States.

You with the Sad Eyes

August 6, 1996, Maui
Pua is the closest thing to perfection that there is. She is the most extraordinary child. I am lifted when I am with her. I am blown away by her magnetism and wisdom. She is a beacon of exuberant light and love. I am so grateful.

When Pua was about three years old, I arrived on the island and rushed to see her — I was so excited, as ever — but as soon as Pua laid eyes on me she glared at me with such disappointment and anger, all haughty and pouty face.

"Hi, Christina *Applegate*," she said. Auntie Kiki had been lying to her all this time.

Pua is in her thirties now, with two kids and a husband. But she still calls me Auntie Kiki.

So no, my name is not Christina Applegate: it's Kiki.

I am a troubled and broken and beautiful and smart and interesting and funny person — I am all the things — but I'm not Christina Applegate. The world puts those two names together and I get the heebie-jeebies.

I'm sorry to my mom and my father, but I reject it.

I hate having to tell people that that's who I am, but when you call me Christina Applegate, you don't fully understand the kind of onus that puts on me.

Christina Applegate is a character, a person who was beholden to people and production companies and everything and everyone else in this town. And she was someone I never was. When I hear that name, I catch my breath, and yet I also don't want the world to fully know who I am either. I suppose this book is a small step to showing you all who I really am.

Actually, a big step.

When I see "Christina Applegate" out in the world—except my star down the hill, goddamn it; I earned that—I always think, *That's a weird name.* Because for my entire life, no one who loves me has called me that. Almost no one—almost no close friends, almost no family—calls me Christina.

When I was growing up, my mom called me Teenybopper.

To his dying day, my father called me Christina.

Being "Christina Applegate" has affected everything.

For a long time, I felt—well, I guess I hoped—that I lived in a magical world where people really loved me for who I was as a person. But stuck here on this MS bed, I've recently been coming to the painful realization that especially when it came to the men in my life, when I met them, they already knew who I was, even if I didn't know who they were. This was especially true during that formative decade I worked on *Married...with Children*. Were men into Kelly Bundy or me?

Recently, this creeping realization has been coming over me: they all knew me. Maybe that's presumptuous to say, but I wonder if I was just a check mark or a fantasy. They could have "Christina Applegate," but they could never have Kiki. I kept her buried deep within. *Married...with Children* was on in ninety or a hundred countries. Later, *Anchorman* was everywhere. *The Sweetest Thing* may have been hated by critics, but it was popular. So much stuff I did meant that I was constantly in the public eye.

Everyone "knew" me before I knew them. What were they thinking? I always wanted to ask, "What were you thinking when you met me? Did you have a preconceived notion of me, and did I disappoint you?" I am not that person that I played, that Christina Applegate from the TV or the movies. I was scrappier, more profane, more romantic, a woman who wrote poetry and desperately wanted to be loved for who she was.

I remember being on a date with someone when I was in my thirties, and I was so excited. We went to the Hotel Bel-Air, to have dinner and drinks. I sat there talking to this guy, being my usual self. We were friends already, but this was the first time we were trying the romantic thing.

But I could see his eyes glassing over, and he was clearly not interested in anything I had to say. I thought I was being cute and funny and flirty.

"Am I bothering you?" I asked. "Do you not want to talk to me?"

"No, no, no. Totally," he said vacantly.

It was evident that I wasn't his cup of tea, and it kind of broke me. Because that happened so many times: people had a preconception of who "Christina Applegate" was—even friends I'd known for a while—and when they met Kiki, they didn't recognize her.

Even thinking about it to this day, it makes me sad. Am I not who people want me to be?

I think I disappointed people, and worse, I don't think they actually wanted to get to know who I really was.

But then you can never live up to something that doesn't exist.

I've always felt like the plus-one in life—not the one invited, but the one who is brought along to make up the numbers. I've never really felt I belong anywhere.

These are the things I think about, lying here on this bed. That feelings spigot—which had been turned off for my entire life because I had to go out and work—is fully open. I'm fifty-three as of this writing and feeling everything, for the first time. I pushed all my feelings down into a Little Ball of Trauma™ in my stomach, but that ball is being pulled apart these days. And the tears feel different, profound, guttural. They're coming from a place that I don't even fully understand.

For so much of my life, I've felt like the good underlies the bad, but something strange has happened, something I'm not used to. I won't lie anymore, be the good girl, and say that any of this is a blessing, but there's some shred of self-understanding that continues to slowly emerge as I tell the story of these past fifty or so years. I want to talk to that little girl who always thought she had to be perfect. Maybe that's what this book is.

All this has left me unable to be polite anymore — it's boring and it takes too much energy. Being kind and loving and nurturing is beautiful, but to be polite is almost to lie. To be respectful is important, but there's something about that sweet politeness demanded of women that stinks of faking our true feelings.

I have done the Superwoman thing once before, after my double mastectomy. I thought I should tell everyone that it was a blessing, when in reality, my body looked like Lorraine Massey, the once beautiful, then grotesque ghost in room 237 at the Overlook Hotel in *The Shining*. I was determined to never do that again. I was going to be honest this time. I hoped

I'd never have to face the choice, but here we are. (Actually, I'm sadder about the mastectomies now when I look down at my body than I was immediately afterward.) With my broken metatarsal, well, a broken bone heals. With the cancer, it was taken out of my body, and I was able to move on.

But MS is my constant companion. In fact, I will probably go away *because* of it. It scares me to death. I don't want to dance with this pain anymore, and I don't want to be in the predicament I'm in. Everything about it sucks.

My knees feel like I have bricks attached to them, heavy and painful. My skin feels like it's got third-degree, fourth-degree, fifth-degree burns. Something is constantly stabbing at my ankles. When I put my feet down on the ground when I wake up, it feels as if the floor is made of needles, yet I can't feel them because my feet are completely numb. Somehow it manages to be both things at once.

All my nerve endings are on fire, sending the wrong signals back to my thirty-lesioned brain. This accounts for the pain I feel twenty-four hours a day. Some days I can get through it, but I'm usually at an eight on the pain scale even if I appear fine. When I walk from my room to Sadie's room, one of my favorite things to do, the pain is almost unbearable—and her room is just down the hallway from mine. And then if (when!) her room isn't picked up, I don't have the balance to get around the things on the floor.

I wish I could say that I am a miracle. Thirty lesions and still kicking. Though most days it's very hard to believe, and in any case, I don't want to minimize what this disease does to a human body and soul. MS is a disease of progression, but it's also a disease of roller coasters. Some days I can bear to dance, others I fear the wheelchair.

That's why *MeSsy,* the podcast I host with my dear friend Jamie-Lynn Sigler, avoids any kind of sugar-coating when it comes to the terrible disease we share. To me, this is part of showing my real self to the world. We've created a sort of MS family through this radical honesty that has led to genuine bright spots, not thoughts and prayers and platitudes. I even met Doug the Pug through the larger MS circle. MS sucks, but the MS community rocks. It took me a long time to lean into that though.

While we were making season 3 of *Dead to Me,* some putrid paparazzo snapped a picture of me in a wheelchair. From there, it was assumed that my character had gotten in an accident, so I had no choice but to announce on social media that I had been diagnosed with multiple sclerosis. I was heartbroken.

The upside is, I think you become a fully human being when people realize you're going through something. I never leave home without my cane. I use it both as a way of not falling and as a barrier. When I carry it, I'm saying, "Nope, don't fuck with me. Don't knock me over. Step back."

Sometimes when a person is in agony it's best to leave them be. My best girlfriend recently went through a horrible tragedy in her life, and at a fundraising party, she turned to me and said, "If one more person looks at me and asks, 'How are you?' — ugh!"

I knew how she felt. On *Dead to Me,* we kept the diagnosis to a small group at first, but eventually everyone knew something was wrong because I was showing up to set in a wheelchair. Finally, I brought the crew together.

"I need you guys to understand that what you've been seeing is actually multiple sclerosis," I said. "And I need you to do me a favor. Please don't ask me how I am in the morning. You can say, 'Hey, bitch!'" A few chuckles rang through the crowd, and I flipped them off as a thank-you. "Anything but 'How are you?' Don't ask me. Because the answer's going to be the same every day: not good. That's how I am."

Across the months, I've become much better at answering the "How are you?" question. It's much easier to answer when you don't worry about what the other person wants to hear.

The true answer is, I'm pissed off. Everything is an effort. Humor disarms the look of concern and pain my friends can't hide when they see me. I don't mind the jokes. Comedy has always been my armor; how else am I going to stop the tears? I don't want to sit here and cry all the time. I have too much to do with what I have left. I am a mother, after all.

Oh, did I mention I wear a diaper? Diapers are very MS chic because many of us have incontinence issues. So fun! But at least they make black ones now. Jamie and I want to start our own diaper line. Each one would have a simple message printed on it:
  FUCK THIS
So if you really want to know how I am: I had to pull shit out of my own ass earlier today because of my disease. Oh, and I fell.

But thank you for asking.

Years ago, I was trying on some pants at Fred Segal, and they were size 2, which is very small. I remember this because usually I was a size 0, and the costume people on *Married... with Children* would often have to take my clothes in. I was bone, bone, bone.

When I looked in a mirror, I saw something no one else saw, but I always did. I worked so hard on my body, but I was never satisfied.

Then I shot *Just Visiting,* the movie where someone on the set had been so cruel to me, in London in 2000.

When we finally wrapped and I'd made it to the airport to go home, I felt like a kidnap victim who had finally been released and was now running toward their family members. I heard later that my friend Jean Reno, who was also in the movie, went into the office of my aggressor and flipped a table on him. In his beautiful French accent, Jean reportedly said, "If I ever zee you treat zomeone like zat again, I'll ferking kill you."

When I got back from London, I got a lot of help for my dysmorphia, even though it would linger. One night, my friends were at my house, and we ordered from Pace, the famous Italian restaurant in the Canyon. They serve a delicious salad called the insalata vegetale. Filled with zucchini, squash, green beans, tomato, garbanzo beans, and olives, it also boasts tons of provolone and fresh mozzarella, as well as being dressed in a red wine vinaigrette. The cheese and the oils were not going in my body, no way, so I asked for no cheese and no dressing. One of my friends, overhearing my order, said "No cheese? But that's the *fun* part!"

Something changed that night. I got it with cheese, and since then, I've never gotten it without. I eat the whole damn delicious thing.

My relationship with food is so much better than it ever was, but it took a long time to improve. It was helped by doing *Sweet Charity,* because to do that show I had to be an athlete. I had to be strong and had to keep up my nutrition.

When the MS hit, the stability I'd fought so hard for went haywire. I had to take fifteen hours of steroid infusions, and immediately everything just went like a fucking blob. It's all documented on the last season of *Dead to Me* and at my Hollywood star ceremony.

By November 2022, when I was to receive my Hollywood Walk of Fame star, I didn't even look like "Christina Applegate" anymore. All the medications and ravages of the disease had loaned me entirely the wrong kind of facelift.

The day I got my star was about the first time anyone had seen me since my diagnosis, and I felt humiliated. I thought I'd even have to go off the rack for the ceremony — and no one goes off the rack in this town — until Christian Siriano came to my rescue and made me something beautiful to wear.

That day I went barefoot because it was too uncomfortable to wear shoes. It's a good job I don't care about germs, though I was a bit worried about stepping on a used needle or something.

Hollywood has seen better times.

The star they gave me is barely a stone's throw from Grauman's Chinese Theatre, right outside the Marshalls on Hollywood and North Orange. That location meant so much to me, to be so central and in the thick of it. I hated how I looked that day, how much this illness had taken from me, but this was my Oscar, after all. It was time to step out in public.

Then something magical happened: a steady, heady stream of my dearest friends went up to the podium and said incredibly lovely things, and by the end of the ceremony, everyone, including me, was crying—even the guy who has to go to all of them because he's the CEO of the whole thing. He said, "I've been to a number of these star ceremonies, and as I sit here and listen to all these tributes, you are by far one of the most beloved recipients of a star that I've ever witnessed."

Damn.

Wouldn't you know it: I'm a survivor yet again.

There's a video of me when they revealed the actual star that day—they had brought me a chair to sit in because...MS—and you can see my feet swinging back and forth like some excited five-and-a-half-year-old in line to see *Star Wars*. *This is magic, this is magic, this is magic...*

Since then, I've sometimes gone down to visit my star in front of Marshalls—say if I have friends in town and they want to see it. I put my mask on and wear the clothes I probably slept in, and we all hang out by the star, just for fun. One time I was sitting by my star, and to make my friends laugh, when tourists would come by and read my name, from behind my mask I'd say, "Oh, it's really sad... she *died*."

For a year or more, people saw only this weird version of me created by those steroid infusions. For all the joy of finally getting my star, it was still humiliating and horrible and devastating to be seen this way. Not just because I was bigger—that was one thing—but because the girl who had control all her life no longer had that control.

I want to throw up when I think of the pictures that are out there of me. I look sad and embarrassed. Because all I can think is, *Everyone is staring.* Once people stared at my boobs; then they stared at my broken foot. But now I knew they were staring not only because I was disabled; they were staring because I was fat, forever an unacceptable fate for women in Hollywood.

"Oh wow," I could imagine everyone saying. "Christina Applegate, of all people, is fat. Not to mention she's got a cane. Not to mention she's got a disease." When I walked out onstage to do Jimmy Kimmel's show three years after my diagnosis, I was touched when Jimmy said, "For people, it's a little bit shocking. You come out with a cane and people love you and are concerned about you." As I told him, this was my now, my normal.

If anyone asks me how I am these days, my answer is always the same: "I'm living the dream, just living *all* the dreams." I use that line because I've found that it curtails people's probing questions.

There was none of me left in that body. The person I'd always been went away and I had to discover who that new person was overnight.

Sometimes the weight bothered me more than the disease. I promised you full honesty, didn't I? I suppose that's the curse of being a woman. Refer back to "mind sticker"; not much has changed.

I didn't look in the mirror for a year.

Then I was put on a clear-liquid diet because of my stomach issues, and all of a sudden, everything just dropped off of me. Within seven months, all of it was gone, and I was down by fifty pounds or more. These days, my legs are tinier than they've ever been.

The illness has given me serious stomach issues. As I write this, there are tamales downstairs that are the best tamales you could ever have—I want to eat five of them right now, I'm so hungry—but I know if I do, I'll probably end up in the ER again, as I have so many times recently. So once again, the good is followed by the bad: I've managed to create a much healthier place when it comes to my relationship with food, only to get out of the shower and see legs that are scary-looking. I have no muscles — just sticks. It's dangerous to be walking around with zero muscles on my body: it means my bones aren't protected if I fall, and it scares me.

But there's still that little voice in my head saying, "You're really skinny. You have the legs you always wanted. Good for you." This is the sickness.

But she's not going to win.

For the longest time, Sadie didn't want to talk about my illness. Even these days, if it comes up, she says, "It's fine."

It's not fine. It has devastated her life.

When she was younger, we had a little pre-bed routine: she'd eat, then we'd dance, then it was bath time, and then I'd read to her. We danced every single night. We called it Dance Party. We'd dance to "I Know What Boys Like" by the Waitresses or "Back in the U.S.S.R." by that guy I kissed that one time.

Sadie has always had a penchant for good music. When she was only five years old, I was in New Orleans shooting *Bad Moms,* and we went down to Bourbon Street to take in the scene. That day we came upon a band busking — bluegrass, delta, jazzy, bluesy stuff, with the washboard and everything — and Sadie couldn't believe what she was seeing. The next thing we knew, she was in the middle of the street, dancing, with her crazy hair that she never wanted brushed. She was really feeling it, so much so that a small crowd formed to watch her. One of the shopkeepers came out with a coffee can and the crowd started putting money in it. She made about thirty dollars, which she then gave to the band.

I fear the Applegate has not fallen far from the tree.

I was a super shy girl — I could never have done what Sadie did that day in New Orleans. But then my mom would remind me that I was on tour with CSNY for years, because of Stephen Stills, and then later with Manassas, because Joe Lala played with them. With Manassas, when they sang "Find the Cost of Freedom," someone in the band would hoist me, then still a baby, like Simba in front of the audiences.

One time we were at a CSN show, and Ringo Starr was there backstage. He asked my mom if he could hold me. But Stephen Stills was my guy, so I punched Ringo a few times and said, "No! I want my Uncle Stephen! I want my Uncle Stephen!"

"Does she not know I'm a fucking Beatle?" Starr reportedly said.

But what I really remember about being on the road was Andy Gibb. Joe Lala played with him, and I was a bit older than in my Simba days, and I can still see the crazy crowds and Andy Gibb taking his shirt off. My babysitter once said, "Christina, why don't you tell Andy what your favorite part of the show is?"

"When you take your shirt off!" I said.

He just laughed in my face. And even as a little girl I knew he didn't love me, didn't want to marry me.

Some days my life hurts so bad that I just sit here and cry—except if Sadie needs me, and I will push through all of it. I'll go to the ends of the earth. Mamas can lift a car, so for her I'm not giving up. Sometimes I want to. Thoughts rush through my head once in a while—bad thoughts. I'm lucky they just pass through. They are thoughts without an object; it's not contemplative in any sense. There's no heaviness to it. They speed away like a douchebag in a Tesla truck.

I've had fun in life, but I'm not sure it was ever happiness, not ever a zephyr that lasted. You can have fun and then everyone leaves, and you're left with yourself and your thoughts and your feelings of loneliness and failure in the world and that overriding fear, "Does anyone really love me? Or will I ever love someone? Will I ever love myself? And why doesn't anyone really know me?" All those questions you have when it's quiet. That's why I always have the TV on: to drown out the noise inside my head. And that's why I'm writing to you now, to tell you who I am, so that at least someone knows before it's too late.

The house in the Canyon, the hit TV shows... those are outside things. I never learned how to deal with the inside parts. I lacked a teacher and couldn't find the truth for myself, but then I remember how often that voice inside my head skews dark. And I remember mornings with my mom, discovering dance, slip-and-sliding with uproarious friends, lying in bed next to my rock god, and of course having my brilliant Sadie. Even all the meditation I did, the time at Agape, those moments of abandon and the moments of freedom—they'd all be taken away by someone hurting me, leaving me here with this huge ball of trauma.

Sylvia, Barbara, Stanley, Meghan Markle, Tootie, Gail, Olivia, Calliope, Stacey, Fucking Bitch... all these body parts letting me down. Though I do talk to them most days, and they listen. Teamwork!

All I ever wanted to do is dance. And be a mother.

As I sit still for the first time in my life, the traumas I buried deep inside rush to the surface and light up like a fireworks display. It's still so beautiful, isn't it?

I know Sadie's heart is broken at what has become of me. One of the ways she deals with it is by making sure that I still mother her. "I want the nachos, but I want them the way Mommy makes them," she'll say. It's her way of getting me to go downstairs, make the snack, and bring it upstairs to her on a tray like my mom used to do for me. All so she can say to herself, "She's still here. She's still my mom and she's still taking care of me."

Yesterday Sadie came and got in my bed and fell asleep on my chest. We had talked a few days earlier about how, just like her mother, she hates being touched, but there she was, asleep on me, holding my hand. I asked her about it later, during one of our "lanai talks" out on the balcony, our sacred Sadie-and-Mama-only time.

"You're my *mom*. I feel safe there," she said.

Sometimes she just reaches over and takes my hand when we're sitting on the bed watching TV. And then if I'm lucky she'll let her eyelids droop...

In fact, she's here right now. I'm typing with one hand. My other hand is tight in hers as she sleeps.

I am Sadie's mother.

I am Kiki.

And that's where I leave you.

ACKNOWLEDGMENTS

Thank you,

To mom. Despite it all you have always been my hero.

To my daily angels. Rachel, Carolyn, Cheryl.

To my "work" angels, as you are so much more to me than that. Thank you for protecting me and loving me. Eric, Rick, Ame, Steve, Huy.

To my book angels. Bryn, who got it; Cindy, who claimed it; L, for it all; Sam, for an author photo I love and so much more.

To my Dutch family. Bram, Nannie, Madea, Nora, Tijmen, Enola. Your love sustains me.

To all my incredible friends who I have known for too many years. Thank you for loving my ugly and still wanting to hang out with me.

To Sean and Marty. I never want to go out with anyone else ever again.

Acknowledgments

To my beloved Jessica, to Jamie and Allison for all of it.
To Marlon. You make life better.
Dad, I miss you.
Tiny, you are one cool papa.
Sadie, every breath is for you.

ABOUT THE AUTHOR

Christina Applegate is an Emmy Award–winning actress known for her captivating performances across film, television, and theatre. With memorable credits including *Anchorman*, *Don't Tell Mom the Babysitter's Dead*, and her Tony-nominated performance in *Sweet Charity* on Broadway, Applegate has solidified her status as a Hollywood legend. In 2024, she launched the *MeSsy* podcast with Jamie-Lynn Sigler about navigating life's curve balls and living with MS. Beyond her success on screen, Applegate is recognized for her advocacy work raising awareness for causes close to her heart. Applegate's talent, grace, and humanitarian work continue to inspire fans worldwide.